The MRI Study Guide for

MW00996035

P 127   good picture of the parts of the magnet. *

Kenneth S. Meacham

The MRI Study Guide
for Technologists

With 51 Illustrations

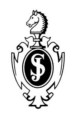

Springer-Verlag
New York Berlin Heidelberg London Paris
Tokyo Hong Kong Barcelona Budapest

Kenneth S. Meacham, R.T. (R), (MR), B.S.
Chief MRI Technologist and MRI Instructor
Atlanta Magnetic Imaging
Atlanta, GA 30342 USA

Library of Congress Cataloging-in-Publication Data
Meacham, Kenneth S.
    The MRI study guide for technologists / Kenneth S. Meacham.
       p.   cm.
    Includes bibliographical references.
    ISBN 0-387-94489-3
    1. Magnetic resonance imaging—Examinations, questions, etc.
  I. Title.
  RC78.7.N83M43   1995
  616.07′548′076—dc20   95-10164

Printed on acid-free paper.

© 1995 Springer-Verlag New York, Inc.
All rights reserved. This work may not be translated or copied in whole or in part without the written permission of the publisher
(Springer-Verlag New York, Inc., 175 Fifth Avenue, New York, NY 10010, USA), except for brief excerpts in connection with
reviews or scholarly analysis. Use in connection with any form of information storage and retrieval, electronic adaptation, computer
software, or by similar or dissimilar methodology now known or hereafter developed is forbidden.
The use of general descriptive names, trade names, trademarks, etc., in this publication, even if the former are not especially
identified, is not to be taken as a sign that such names, as understood by the Trade Marks and Merchandise Marks Act, may
accordingly be used freely by anyone.
While the advice and information in this book are believed to be true and accurate at the date of going to press, neither the authors
nor the editors nor the publisher can accept any legal responsibility for any errors or omissions that may be made. The publisher
makes no warranty, express or implied, with respect to the material contained herein.

Production managed by Hal Henglein; manufacturing supervised by Jacqui Ashri.
Camera-ready copy prepared by the author.
Printed and bound by Maple-Vail, York, PA.
Printed in the United States of America.

9 8 7 6 5 4 3 2 1

ISBN 0-387-94489-3 Springer-Verlag New York Berlin Heidelberg

To my wife Beverly
for her love and support

Preface

It has been said many times over that practice is the best way to prepare for any event that one wants to complete successfully. Whether it is a football game, a chess match, or an examination, good preparation involves practice. Thorough preparation for any event increases confidence, reduces anxiety, and heightens one's ability to succeed. Because it is the MRI registry that we are preparing for, this book has been written in a practice format for technologists. The areas covered in this book are basic to MRI and are non-manufacturer specific with the exception of some of the parameter terms. Throughout the book many of the different terms used to describe a single principle have been used with the hopes of preparing the technologist for any way a question may be worded. With the exception of the cross sectional anatomy section, the answers to each question have been included on the same page to increase learning efficiency but they are also easy to hide so that testing one's knowledge can also be achieved. The correct answer to each question is always within the selection. The books within the bibliography are all excellent for technologists and are highly recommended for increasing one's understanding of magnetic resonance imaging. I have worked diligently to assure that this book is thorough and I sincerely hope that it will be the tool that provides the highest level of preparation. **GOOD LUCK!**

Kenneth S. Meacham

Acknowledgments

When I began this project I never knew the amount of work that it would take to complete, and without the help of many great people this book would not exist. I would first like to thank Mike Perry for continually working to motivate me and for critically evaluating every step. I would also like to thank Fred Chitwood, Paul Woodard, Kristine Porter, Aileen Mains, and Dr. John Bisese for their help and inspiration.

Contents

SECTION 1

History

Magnetism
MRI

1. The area in Asia Minor that first discovered magnets is known as_____.
    A. Rumania
    B. Magnesia
    C. Magnomia
    D. None of the above

2. The first magnets were called Magnetites because the people that lived in the area where they were found were known as _____.
    A. Magnesians
    B. Magnomians
    C. Magnetes
    D. None of the above

3. For centuries, sailors used magnets for which of the following purposes?
    A. Lift heavy objects
    B. Navigate the seas
    C. Pull up anchors
    D. None of the above

4. Which of the following people named the ends of a magnet north and south poles?
    A. Louis Faraday
    B. Alexander Necham
    C. Petrus Peregtinus de Maricourt
    D. Hans Christian

5. In 1825, the British scientist, William Surgeon, constructed the first _____.
    A. Superconducting magnet
    B. Permanent magnet
    C. Electromagnet
    D. None of the above

1.b 2.c 3.b 4.c 5.c

6. The law of magnetic induction that is used in MRI today was developed by which of the following people?
   A. Wilhelm Weber
   B. Michael Faraday
   C. Hans Christian
   D. Albert Einstein

7. The first magnetic resonance experiments with liquids were conducted by a group of scientists from Stanford University led by which of the following people?
   A. Felix Bloch
   B. Edward Purcell
   C. Otto Stern
   D. Paul Lauterbur

8. The first magnetic resonance experiments with solids were conducted by a group of scientists from Harvard University led by which of the following people?
   A. Felix Bloch
   B. Edward Purcell
   C. Otto Stern
   D. Paul Lauterbur

9. Which of the following people won the 1952 Nobel Prize for their NMR research?
   A. Felix Bloch
   B. I.I. Rabi
   C. Edward Purcell
   D. Both A and C

10. Scientist Paul Lauterbur described an NMR imaging technique called _____.
   A. Magnetography
   B. Positron Tomography
   C. Zeugmatography
   D. Computed Tomography

6.b 7.a 8.b 9.d 10.c

11. Which of the following people produced the first crude MRI image showing a rat tumor, which later appeared on the cover of *Science* magazine?
    A. Paul Lauterbur
    B. Raymond Damadian
    C. Felix Bloch
    D. Edward Purcell

12. The first whole body MRI scanner used by Dr. Raymond Damadian was known as the _____.
    A. Signa
    B. Gyroscan
    C. Indomitable
    D. Abominable

13. The word lodestone was derived from which of the following meanings?
    A. Attraction
    B. To find one's way
    C. Heavy
    D. None of the above

14. Which of the following people was attributed in 1967 with producing the first MR signals from a live animal?
    A. Edward Purcell
    B. Felix Bloch
    C. Paul Lauterbur
    D. Jasper Jackson

15. The magnetic properties of the nucleus of atoms were discovered in 1924 by which of the following people?
    A. Edward Purcell
    B. Raymond Damadian
    C. Joseph Henry
    D. Wolfgang Pauli

11.b 12.c 13.b 14.d 15.d
A

16. The first MRI images of a human were obtained in what year?
    A. 1929
    B. 1977
    C. 1983
    D. 1944

17. The magnet's ability to attract and repel objects was first described by which of the following people?
    A. Alexander Necham
    B. Lucretius Cerus
    C. Hoang-ti
    D. None of the above

18. The first whole body MRI scanner was a superconductive magnet with a field strength of _____.
    A. 3000 gauss
    B. 5000 gauss
    C. 10000 gauss
    D. 15000 gauss

19. The first whole body MRI scanner was constructed at which of the following facilities?
    A. Harvard University Medical Center
    B. Stanford University Medical Center
    C. Yale University Medical Center
    D. Downstate Medical Center, New York

20. Dr. Raymond Damadian was inducted into the National Inventors Hall of Fame for his invention of the first human scanner in what year?
    A. 1974
    B. 1978
    C. 1982
    D. 1989

16.b 17.b 18.b 19.d 20.d

21. Which of the following people developed the most effective way to generate and transmit alternating current and has a magnetic unit of measurement named after him?
    A. Michael Faraday
    B. Nikola Tesla
    C. Niels Bohr
    D. Jean Baptiste Joseph Fourier

22. Which of the following people developed the complex mathematical formulas used in MRI to reconstruct signals into images?
    A. Michael Faraday
    B. Nikola Tesla
    C. Niels Bohr
    D. Jean Baptiste Joseph Fourier

23. Which of the following people received the 1922 Nobel prize in physics for his theory of the atomic structure?
    A. Michael Faraday
    B. Nikola Tesla
    C. Niels Bohr
    D. Otto Stern

24. Which of the following people received the 1943 Nobel prize in physics for his development of a method to study the magnetic moments of atoms by directing atomic beams through magnetic fields?
    A. Nikola Tesla
    B. Thomas Edison
    C. Otto Stern
    D. Niels Bohr

21.b 22.d 23.c 24.c

Match the scientist with his contribution to MRI by placing the letter that corresponds to the scientist in the box next to his accomplishment.

A. Jean Baptiste Joseph Fourier   **E.** Felix Bloch

B. Michael Faraday   **F.** Edward Purcell

C. Niels Bohr   **G.** Paul Lauterbur

D. Nikola Tesla   **H.** Raymond Damadian

☐ Won the 1952 Nobel Prize for NMR research

☐ Developed the mathematical formula used to reconstruct images from signal

☐ Described the imaging technique known as Zeugmatography

☐ Discovered the law of magnetic induction

☐ Developed the theory of atomic structure

☐ Designed the first whole body NMR scanner for imaging

☐ Developed a method to generate alternating current and has a magnetic unit of measurement named after him

SECTION 2

Basic Principles

Atomic Structure
Basic Magnetism
Nuclear Magnetism
Alignment
Precession
Resonance
Relaxation
Signal Production
Timing Parameters

1. With the exception of hydrogen, all matter is composed of three components.
    They are _____.
    A. Electrons, Photons, Protons
    B. Electrons, Neutrons, Photons
    C. Protons, Neutrons, Photons
    D. Neutrons, Electrons, Protons

2. The positively charged component of an atom is called the _____.
    A. Electron
    B. Proton
    C. Positron
    D. Neutron

3. The negatively charged component of an atom is called the _____.
    A. Electron
    B. Proton
    C. Negatron
    D. Neutron

4. The neutral component of an atom is called the _____.
    A. Electron
    B. Proton
    C. Neutron
    D. Photon

5. The nucleus of the hydrogen atom is made up of one _____.
    A. Neutron
    B. Electron
    C. Photon
    D. Proton

6. Materials reach their highest magnetic potential when their atoms are grouped
    in areas known as _____.
    A. Regions
    B. Fields
    C. Fringes
    D. Domains

1.d 2.b 3.a 4.c 5.d 6.d

7. Material that is weakly attracted to a magnetic field is said to be _____.
    A. Electromagnetic
    B. Paramagnetic
    C. Ferromagnetic
    D. Diamagnetic

8. Material that is strongly attracted to a magnetic field is said to be _____.
    A. Electromagnetic
    B. Paramagnetic
    C. Ferromagnetic
    D. Diamagnetic

9. Material that is slightly repelled from a magnetic field is said to be _____.
    A. Resistive
    B. Paramagnetic
    C. Ferromagnetic
    D. Diamagnetic

10. Three types of ferromagnetic material are _____.
    A. Copper, Titanium, Aluminum
    B. Iron, Cobalt, Nickel
    C. Bronze, Niobium, Tin
    D. None of the above

11. To exist, magnets must have two poles, therefore they are commonly called
    _____.
    A. Vectors
    B. Dipoles
    C. Axis
    D. Both A and C

12. The lines that represent the field of a magnet are known as _____.
    A. Flux lines
    B. Intensity lines
    C. Induction lines
    D. Faraday lines

7.b 8.c 9.d 10.b 11.b 12.a

13. The strength of a magnet is measured by its _____.
    A. Signal intensity
    B. Induction ability
    C. Flux density
    D. None of the above

14. The strength of an MRI magnet is most commonly represented by a unit of measurement called _____.
    A. Amps
    B. Kilogauss
    C. Tesla
    D. Ohms

15. 10,000 gauss is equal to _____.
    A. 1.0 amp
    B. 1.0 ohm
    C. 1.0 tesla
    D. 10 tesla

16. 15,000 gauss is equal to _____.
    A. 1.5 amps
    B. 1.5 ohms
    C. 1.5 tesla
    D. 15 tesla

17. The law that is used in MRI to describe how a magnetic field is induced by flowing current is known as _____.
    A. Damadian's Law
    B. Murphy's Law
    C. Newton's Law
    D. Faraday's Law

18. Which of the following is an advantage of a permanent magnet MRI system?
    A. Very heavy
    B. Low operating costs
    C. Fixed field strength

13.c 14.c 15.c 16.c 17.d 18.b

19. What type of molecule makes up 50% to 90% of a person's total body weight?
    A. Fat
    B. Oxygen
    C. Water
    D. Nitrogen

20. Clinical MRI is based on the generation of signal from the nucleus of which atom?
    A. Helium
    B. Nitrogen
    C. Oxygen
    D. Hydrogen

21. The nucleus of the hydrogen atom carries what type of charge?
    A. Negative
    B. Neutral
    C. Positive

22. The spin of the proton of the hydrogen atom is known as _____.
    A. Nuclear spin
    B. Axial momentum
    C. Hydraulic spin
    D. Angular momentum

23. Because the nucleus of the hydrogen atom acts much like a bar magnet it is said to have a _____.
    A. Magnetic ratio
    B. Magnetic moment
    C. Larmor ratio
    D. Frequency ratio

24. Because the spinning nucleus of the hydrogen atom has both a North and South pole it is commonly called a _____.
    A. Electromagnet
    B. Bar magnet
    C. Dipole

19.c 20.d 21.c 22.d 23.b 24.c

25. When placed in an external magnetic field, hydrogen nuclei _____.
    A. Resonate
    B. Become excited
    C. Become aligned
    D. Repel each other

26. After being placed in an external magnetic field, high energy hydrogen nuclei point in which direction?
    A. Parallel
    B. Anti-paired
    C. Anti-parallel
    D. Perpendicular

27. After being placed in an external magnetic field, low energy hydrogen nuclei point in which direction?
    A. Parallel
    B. Anti-paired
    C. Anti-parallel
    D. Perpendicular

28. When placed in an external magnetic field, the hydrogen nuclei that are of clinical interest are _____.
    A. Parallel paired
    B. Anti-parallel paired
    C. Parallel unpaired
    D. Perpendicular paired

29. When a patient is placed in an external magnetic field, the number of unmatched hydrogen protons usually equals _____.
    A. One billion
    B. One million
    C. Few per million
    D. Few per billion

25.c 26.c 27.a 28.c 29.c

30. The sum of all of the unmatched parallel protons in an external magnetic field makes up what is called the _____.
    A. External magnetization
    B. Internal magnetization
    C. Resonant magnetization
    D. Net magnetic vector

31. The type of rotation that is displayed by hydrogen nuclei in an external magnetic field is known as _____.
    A. Magnetization
    B. Relaxation
    C. Precession
    D. Resonance

32. Within a perfect magnetic field all protons rotate at _____.
    A. Different frequencies
    B. The same frequency
    C. Undetermined frequencies
    D. None of the above

33. The speed at which protons rotate in an external magnetic field is known as _____.
    A. Precessional frequency
    B. Hydromagnetic frequency
    C. External magnetic frequency
    D. None of the above

34. The ratio that describes the constant at which any magnetic nucleus will precess in a 1 tesla magnet is known as _____.
    A. Precessional ratio
    B. Magnetogyric ratio
    C. Gyromagnetic ratio
    D. Both B and C

30.d 31.c 32.b 33.a 34.d

35. The precessional frequency of magnetic nuclei is determined by which of the following ?
    A. The strength of the external magnetic field
    B. The magnetogyric frequency
    C. The gyromagnetic ratio of the specific nuclei
    D. Both A and C

36. The equation that is used to determine the precessional frequency of magnetic nuclei is known as _____.
    A. Faraday's equation
    B. Fast Fourier transformations
    C. Damadian's equation
    D. Larmor equation

37. The stronger the magnetic field the_____ the precessional frequency.
    A. Stronger
    B. Higher
    C. Longer
    D. Shorter

38. Which of the following is the equation that is used to determine precessional frequencies?
    A. Wo = yBo
    B. Bo = yWo
    C. F = yBo
    D. Both A and C

39. Alignment of the net magnetic vector in the direction of the external magnetic field is known as _____.
    A. Transverse magnetization
    B. Longitudinal magnetization
    C. Equilibrium
    D. Both B and C

35.d 36.d 37.b 38.d 39.d

40. Magnetization in the XY plane is known as _____.
    A. Equilibrium
    B. Longitudinal magnetization
    C. Transverse magnetization
    D. Spin-Lattice magnetization

41. When the proper radio frequency is applied, the precessing hydrogen nuclei begin to _____.
    A. Dephase
    B. Rephase
    C. Relax
    D. Resonate

42. The RF pulse used to move nuclei into a higher energy state is at a frequency known as _____.
    A. Resonance frequency
    B. Fourier frequency
    C. Transverse frequency
    D. None of the above

43. Hydrogen nuclei begin to precess in phase when which of the following occurs?
    A. The proper RF is turned off
    B. The patient is placed into the external magnet
    C. The proper RF is turned on
    D. None of the above

44. When the radio frequency is turned off, precessing nuclei begin to _____.
    A. Relax
    B. Lose energy
    C. Dephase
    D. All of the above

40.c 41.d 42.a 43.c 44.d

45. Another name for transverse relaxation is _____.
    A. Spin-Lattice relaxation
    B. T1 relaxation
    C. Spin-Spin relaxation
    D. Longitudinal relaxation

46. Another name for T1 relaxation is _____.
    A. Dephasing
    B. Longitudinal relaxation
    C. Spin-Spin relaxation
    D. Transverse relaxation

47. The return of longitudinal magnetization to equilibrium is known as _____.
    A. T1 relaxation
    B. Spin-Lattice relaxation
    C. Longitudinal relaxation
    D. All of the above

48. Dephasing of the net vector in the transverse plane is known as _____.
    A. T1 relaxation
    B. Spin-Lattice relaxation
    C. Longitudinal relaxation
    D. Spin-Spin relaxation

49. The time it takes for a tissue's bulk longitudinal magnetization to return to 63% of its original value is known as _____.
    A. T1 relaxation time
    B. T2 relaxation time
    C. T2* relaxation time
    D. None of the above

45.c 46.b 47.d 48.d 49.a

50. The time it takes for transverse magnetization to decay to 37% of its original value is known as _____.
    A. T1 relaxation time
    B. T2 relaxation time
    C. T2* relaxation time

51. Dephasing of the net vector in the transverse plane is caused by two factors, imperfections in the external magnetic field and _____.
    A. The application of the 180 degree RF pulse
    B. The application of a 90 degree RF pulse
    C. Interaction between surrounding nuclei
    D. None of the above

52. Magnetization in the transverse plane can also be known as _____.
    A. Mz
    B. Mxy
    C. Mo
    D. Both B and C

53. Magnetization in the longitudinal plane can also be known as _____.
    A. Mz
    B. Equilibrium
    C. Mxy
    D. Both A and B

54. MRI signals can only be detected in which of the following planes?
    A. Z plane
    B. XY plane
    C. Transverse plane
    D. Both B and C

50.b 51.c 52.d 53.d 54.d

55. The signal created after applying a 90 degree RF pulse is known as a _____.
    A. Gradient echo signal
    B. Spin echo signal
    C. Spin spin signal
    D. FID Signal

56. The signal produced after the 180 degree RF pulse is applied is known as a
    _____ .
    A. Gradient echo signal
    B. Spin echo signal
    C. Spin spin signal
    D. FID signal

57. A 180 degree RF pulse is used to _____ the dephasing net vector in the transverse plane.
    A. Magnetize
    B. Decay
    C. Delay
    D. Refocus

58. The larger the net magnetic vector in the transverse plane the _____ the signal that is produced.
    A. Smaller
    B. Stronger
    C. Weaker
    D. None of the above

59. The smaller the net magnetic vector in the transverse plane the _____ the signal that is produced.
    A. Larger
    B. Stronger
    C. Weaker
    D. None of the above

55.d 56.b 57.d 58.b 59.c

60. The letters FID in an FID signal stand for _____.
   A. Field image dimensions
   B. Free induction decay
   C. Field induction direction
   D. Free image direction

61. The type of signal that is created after a gradient is used to refocus the dephasing net vector is known as _____.
   A. Spin echo signal
   B. Gradient echo signal
   C. FID signal
   D. None of the above

62. The time between two successive 90 degree RF pulses is known as _____.
   A. Echo time
   B. Repetition time
   C. Inversion time
   D. Relaxation time

63. The time between the 90 degree RF pulse and the spin echo signal in a spin echo pulse sequence is known as _____.
   A. Echo time
   B. Repetition time
   C. Inversion time
   D. Relaxation time

64. In an inversion recovery pulse sequence, the time between the 180 degree RF pulse and the 90 degree RF pulse is known as _____.
   A. Echo time
   B. Repetition time
   C. Inversion time
   D. Relaxation time

60.b 61.b 62.b 63.a 64.c

A. _____

B. _____

C. _____

With the information given, label each atomic particle.

Tesla	Gauss
.3	
.5	
1.0	
1.5	
2.0	

Using the correct answer to question 15, convert each field strength from tesla to gauss.

Field Strength	Gyromagnetic Ratio	Precessional Frequency
.3	42.6	
.5	42.6	
1.0	42.6	
1.5	42.6	
2.0	42.6	

Using the Larmor equation, calculate the precessional frequency of hydrogen at each field strength.

$$F=yBo$$

F = Precessional Frequency
y = Gyromagnetic Ratio
Bo = Field Strength

SECTION 3

Image Weighting and Contrast

T1 Contrast
T2 Contrast
Proton Density Contrast
T2* Decay
Tissue Relaxation Times
Tissue Relaxation Charts

1. MRI images that are based on the differences in longitudinal relaxation characteristics of tissues are known as _____.
     A. T1 weighted images
     B. T2 weighted images
     C. Proton density weighted images
     D. Transitional images

2. MRI images that are based on the differences in the amount of hydrogen nuclei in tissues are known as _____.
     A. T1 weighted images
     B. T2 weighted images
     C. Proton density weighted images
     D. Transitional images

3. MRI images that are based on the differences in the transverse relaxation characteristics of tissues are known as _____.
     A. T1 weighted images
     B. T2 weighted images
     C. Proton density weighted images
     D. Spin density weighted images

4. The image parameter that primarily affects T1 weighting is _____.
     A. Echo time
     B. Inversion time
     C. Repetition time
     D. None of the above

5. The image parameter that primarily affects T2 weighting is _____.
     A. Echo time
     B. Inversion time
     C. Repetition time
     D. None of the above

1.a 2.c 3.b 4.c 5.a

6. In a T1 weighted image, a short TR is used to _____.
    A. Maximize T2 effects
    B. Minimize T2 effects
    C. Maximize T1 effects
    D. Minimize T1 effects

7. In a T2 weighted image, a long TR is used to _____.
    A. Maximize T2 effects
    B. Minimize T2 effects
    C. Maximize T1 effects
    D. Minimize T1 effects

8. In a T2 weighted image, a long TE is used to _____.
    A. Maximize T2 effects
    B. Minimize T2 effects
    C. Maximize T1 effects
    D. Minimize T1 effects

9. In a T1 weighted image, a short TE is used to _____.
    A. Maximize T2 effects
    B. Minimize T2 effects
    C. Maximize T1 effects
    D. Minimize T1 effects

10. In a T1 weighted image, tissues with short T1 relaxation times produce what type of signal?
    A. High
    B. Low
    C. Intermediate
    D. None of the above

6.c 7.d 8.a 9.b 10.a

11. In a T1 weighted image, tissues with long T1 relaxation times produce what type of signal?
    A. High
    B. Low
    C. Intermediate
    D. None of the above

12. In a T2 weighted image, tissues with short T2 relaxation times appear _____.
    A. Hyperintense
    B. Hypointense
    C. Isointense
    D. None of the above

13. In a T2 weighted image, tissues with long T2 relaxation times appear _____.
    A. Hyperintense
    B. Hypointense
    C. Isointense
    D. None of the above

14. In a proton density weighted image, tissues with a high number of hydrogen nuclei appear _____.
    A. Hyperintense
    B. Hypointense
    C. Isointense
    D. None of the above

15. In a proton density weighted image, tissues with a low number of hydrogen nuclei appear _____.
    A. Hyperintense
    B. Hypointense
    C. Isointense
    D. None of the above

11.b 12.b 13.a 14.a 15.b

16. In biological tissue, which type of relaxation occurs the quickest?
    A. T2 relaxation
    B. T2* relaxation
    C. T1 relaxation
    D. None of the above

17. Longitudinal relaxation occurs more efficiently in which type of tissue?
    A. Water
    B. Fat
    C. Muscle
    D. Cortical bone

18. In a T1 weighted image, fat has a _____ T1 relaxation time and therefore appears_____.
    A. Long, Bright
    B. Long, Dark
    C. Short, Dark
    D. Short, Bright

19. In a T1 weighted image, CSF has a _____ T1 relaxation time and therefore appears_____.
    A. Long, Bright
    B. Long, Dark
    C. Short, Dark
    D. Short, Bright

20. In a T2 weighted image, fat has a _____ T2 relaxation time and therefore appears_____.
    A. Long, Bright
    B. Long, Dark
    C. Short, Dark
    D. Short, Bright

16.b 17.a 18.d 19.b 20.c

See p. 20 top. 6 page
mRIP 4 p19

21. In a T2 weighted image, CSF has a _____ T2 relaxation time and therefore appears _____.
    A. Long, Bright
    B. Long, Dark
    C. Short, Dark
    D. Short, Bright

22. A spin echo image with a long TR and a short TE is known as what type of image?
    A. T1 weighted image
    B. Proton density weighted image
    C. Spin density weighted image
    D. Both B and C

23. A spin echo image with a long TR and a long TE is known as what type of image?
    A. T1 weighted image
    B. Proton density weighted image
    C. T2 weighted image
    D. Spin density weighted image

24. A spin echo image with a short TR and a short TE is known as what type of image?
    A. T1 weighted image
    B. T2 weighted image
    C. Proton density weighted image
    D. None of the above

25. Another name for a proton density weighted image is _____.
    A. Spin density
    B. Intermediate
    C. Inversion recovery
    D. Both A and B

21.a 22.d 23.c 24.a 25.d

26. On a T1 weighted image of the brain, fat appears_____ to white matter.
    A. Hyperintense
    B. Hypointense
    C. Isointense

27. On a T1 weighted image of the brain, white matter appears_____ to grey matter.
    A. Hyperintense
    B. Hypointense
    C. Isointense

28. On a T1 weighted image of the brain, grey matter appears_____ to CSF.
    A. Hyperintense
    B. Hypointense
    C. Isointense

29. On a T1 weighted image of the brain, CSF appears_____ to fat.
    A. Hyperintense
    B. Hypointense
    C. Isointense

30. On a proton density weighted image of the brain, white matter appears_____ to grey matter.
    A. Hyperintense
    B. Hypointense
    C. Isointense

31. On a proton density weighted image of the brain, CSF appears_____ to grey matter.
    A. Hyperintense
    B. Hypointense
    C. Isointense

26.a 27.a 28.a 29.b 30.b 31.b

32. On a T2 weighted image of the brain, CSF appears _____ to grey matter.
    A. Hyperintense
    B. Hypointense
    C. Isointense

33. On a T2 weighted image of the brain, grey matter appears_____ to white matter.
    A. Hyperintense
    B. Hypointense
    C. Isointense

34. On a T1 weighted image of the knee, cortical bone appears _____ to all other tissues.
    A. Hyperintense
    B. Hypointense
    C. Isointense

35. On a T1 weighted image of the knee, bone marrow appears _____ to meniscal tissues.
    A. Hyperintense
    B. Hypointense
    C. Isointense

36. On a T1 weighted image of the spine, the intervertebral disk appears_____ to spinal cord.
    A. Hyperintense
    B. Hypointense
    C. Isointense

32.a 33.a 34.b 35.a 36.b

37. On a T2 weighted image of the spine, the intervertebral disk appears _____ to the spinal cord.
    A. Hyperintense
    B. Hypointense
    C. Isointense

38. At a field strength of 1.0 tesla, the approximate T1 relaxation time of fat is _____.
    A. 180 ms
    B. 270 ms
    C. 360 ms
    D. 390 ms

39. At a field strength of 1.0 tesla, the approximate T2 relaxation time of fat is _____.
    A. 40 ms
    B. 50 ms
    C. 80 ms
    D. 90 ms

40. At a field strength of 1.0 tesla, the approximate T1 relaxation time of liver tissue is _____.
    A. 180 ms
    B. 270 ms
    C. 360 ms
    D. 390 ms

41. At a field strength of 1.0 tesla, the approximate T2 relaxation time of liver tissue is _____.
    A. 40 ms
    B. 50 ms
    C. 60 ms
    D. 70 ms

37.a 38.a 39.d 40.b 41.b

42. At a field strength of 1.0 tesla, the approximate T1 relaxation time for spleen tissue is _____.
    A. 360 ms
    B. 380 ms
    C. 400 ms
    D. 480 ms

43. At a field strength of 1.0 tesla, the approximate T2 relaxation time for spleen tissue is _____.
    A. 60 ms
    B. 80 ms
    C. 90 ms
    D. 100 ms

44. At a field strength of 1.0 tesla, the approximate T1 relaxation time for grey matter is _____.
    A. 390 ms
    B. 450 ms
    C. 520 ms
    D. 620 ms

45. At a field strength of 1.0 tesla, the approximate T2 relaxation time for grey matter is _____.
    A. 70 ms
    B. 80 ms
    C. 90 ms
    D. 100 ms

46. At a field strength of 1.0 tesla, the approximate T1 relaxation time for white matter is _____.
    A. 180 ms
    B. 270 ms
    C. 360 ms
    D. 390 ms

42.d 43.b 44.c 45.d 46.d

47. At a field strength of 1.0 tesla, the approximate T2 relaxation time for white matter is _____.
    A. 80 ms
    B. 90 ms
    C. 100 ms
    D. 140 ms

48. At a field strength of 1.0 tesla, the approximate T1 relaxation time for renal cortex tissue is _____.
    A. 180 ms
    B. 270 ms
    C. 360 ms
    D. 390 ms

49. At a field strength of 1.0 tesla, the approximate T2 relaxation time for renal cortex tissue is _____.
    A. 45 ms
    B. 50 ms
    C. 60 ms
    D. 70 ms

50. At a field strength of 1.0 tesla, the approximate T1 relaxation time for muscle tissue is _____.
    A. 270 ms
    B. 480 ms
    C. 600 ms
    D. 680 ms

51. At a field strength of 1.0 tesla, the approximate T2 relaxation time for muscle tissue is _____.
    A. 40 ms
    B. 70 ms
    C. 80 ms
    D. 100 ms

47.b 48.c 49.d 50.c 51.a

52. At a field strength of 1.0 tesla, the approximate T1 relaxation time for renal medulla tissue is _____.
    A. 520 ms
    B. 600 ms
    C. 680 ms
    D. 800 ms

53. At a field strength of 1.0 tesla, the approximate T2 relaxation time for renal medulla tissue is _____.
    A. 90 ms
    B. 100 ms
    C. 140 ms
    D. 300 ms

54. At a field strength of 1.0 tesla, the approximate T1 relaxation time for blood is _____.
    A. 540 ms
    B. 680 ms
    C. 800 ms
    D. 1000 ms

55. At a field strength of 1.0 tesla, the approximate T2 relaxation time for blood is _____.
    A. 140 ms
    B. 180 ms
    C. 240 ms
    D. 300 ms

56. At a field strength of 1.0 tesla, the approximate T1 relaxation time for CSF is _____.
    A. 800 ms
    B. 1000 ms
    C. 2000 ms
    D. 2500 ms

52.c 53.c 54.c 55.b 56.c

57. At a field strength of 1.0 tesla, the approximate T2 relaxation time for CSF is
_____.
   A. 70 ms
   B. 100 ms
   C. 180 ms
   D. 300 ms

58. At a field strength of 1.0 tesla, the approximate T1 relaxation time for water
is _____.
   A. 800 ms
   B. 1000 ms
   C. 2000 ms
   D. 2500 ms

59. At a field strength of 1.0 tesla, the approximate T2 relaxation time for water
is _____.
   A. 800 ms
   B. 1000 ms
   C. 2000 ms
   D. 2500 ms

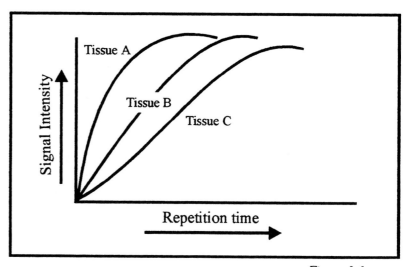

Figure 3-1

60. Figure 3-1 displays which type of relaxation curve?
   A. T1 Relaxation curve
   B. T2 relaxation curve
   C. Inversion recovery curve

57.d 58.d 59.d 60.a

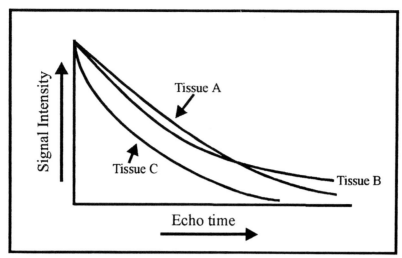

Figure 3-2

61. Figure 3-2 displays which type of relaxation curve?
   A. T1 relaxation curve
   B. T2 relaxation curve
   C. Inversion recovery curve

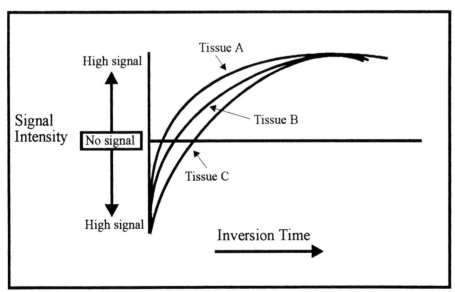

Figure 3-3

61.b

62. Figure 3-3 displays which type of relaxation curve?
 A. T1 relaxation curve
 B. T2 relaxation curve
 C. Inversion recovery curve

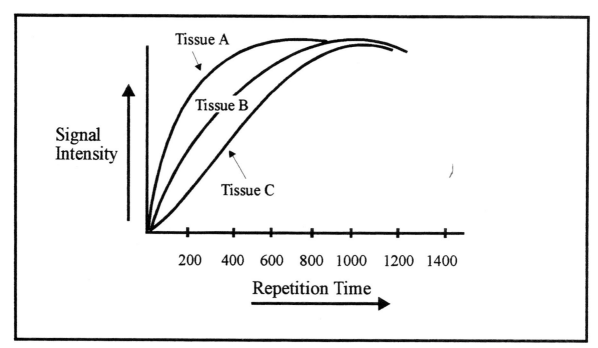

Figure 3-4

63. In Figure 3-4, at a TR of 200, which of the following tissues has the greatest signal intensity?
 A. Tissue A
 B. Tissue B
 C. Tissue C

62.c 63.a

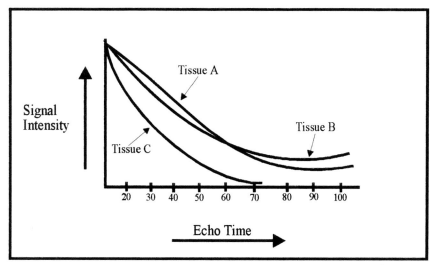

Figure 3-5

64. In figure 3-5, at a TE of 90, which of the following tissues has the greatest signal intensity?
   A. Tissue A
   B. Tissue B
   C. Tissue C

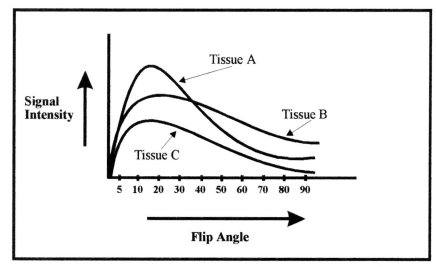

Figure 3-6

65. Figure 3-6 displays which type of relaxation curve?
   A. T1 relaxation curve
   B. Inversion recovery curve
   C. T2 relaxation curve
   D. T2* relaxation curve

64.b 65.d

In section 3, using the correct answers to questions 38 through 59, fill in the tissue relaxation chart.

Approximate Relaxation Times at 1.0 Tesla

Tissue	T1 time	T2 time
Fat		
Liver		
Renal cortex		
White matter		
Spleen		
Grey matter		
Muscle		
Renal medulla		
Blood		
CSF		
Water		

SECTION 4

Image Production

Gradients
Spacial Encoding
Fourier Transformation
K Space
Image Quality
Image Parameters
Image Acquisition

1. The precessional frequency of hydrogen at 1.5 tesla is _____.
   A. 42.6 MHz
   B. 63.86 MHz
   C. 63.86 KHz
   D. 21.28 KHz

2. The precessional frequency of hydrogen at 1.0 tesla is _____.
   A. 42.6 MHz
   B. 63.86 MHz
   C. 25.48 MHz
   D. 21.28 KHz

3. The precessional frequency of hydrogen at .5 tesla is _____.
   A. 42.6 MHz
   B. 63.86 MHz
   C. 25.48 MHz
   D. 21.28 MHz

4. The coils used to alter the magnetic field during scanning are known as the

   _____.
   A. RF receive coils
   B. RF transmit coils
   C. Shim coils
   D. Gradient coils

5. The precessional frequency of hydrogen nuclei that experience increased magnetic field strength due to gradient coils _____.
   A. Increases
   B. Decreases
   C. Stays the same

6. The precessional frequency of hydrogen nuclei that experience decreased magnetic field strength due to gradient coils _____.
   A. Increases
   B. Decreases
   C. Stays the same

1.b 2.a 3.d 4.d 5.a 6.b

7. There are how many pairs of gradient coils in a standard MRI system?
  A. 1 pair
  B. 2 pairs
  C. 3 pairs
  D. 4 pairs

8. The Z gradient alters the magnetic field strength along which axis?
  A. Horizontal axis
  B. Vertical axis
  C. Long axis
  D. Short axis

9. The Y gradient alters the magnetic field strength along which axis?
  A. Horizontal axis
  B. Vertical axis
  C. Long axis
  D. Short axis

10. The X gradient alters the magnetic field strength along which axis?
  A. Horizontal axis
  B. Vertical axis
  C. Long axis
  D. Short axis

11. The center of the magnet where the magnetic field strength remains unchanged even during the application of gradient magnetic fields is known as the _____.
  A. Pericenter
  B. Isocenter
  C. Monocenter
  D. None of the above

7.c 8.c 9.b 10.a 11.b

12. The three primary functions that gradients perform during MR scanning are_____.
   A. Slice selection, RF application, Frequency encoding
   B. Phase encoding, Frequency encoding, RF application
   C. Slice selection, Phase encoding, Frequency encoding
   D. None of the above

13. During slice selection, the Z gradient is used to select slices in which plane?
   A. Coronal
   B. Axial
   C. Sagittal
   D. None of the above

14. During slice selection, the X gradient is used to select slices in which plane?
   A. Coronal
   B. Axial
   C. Sagittal
   D. None of the above

15. During slice selection, the Y gradient is used to select slices in which plane?
   A. Coronal
   B. Axial
   C. Sagittal
   D. None of the above

16. During the acquisition of sagittal images with the frequency direction S/I, phase encoding is conducted by which physical gradient?
   A. X gradient
   B. Y gradient
   C. Z gradient
   D. None of the above

12.c 13.b 14.c 15.a 16.b

17. During the acquisition of coronal images with the frequency direction S/I, phase encoding is conducted by which physical gradient?
    A. X gradient
    B. Y gradient
    C. Z gradient
    D. None of the above

18. During the acquisition of axial images of the brain with the frequency direction A/P, phase encoding is performed by which physical gradient?
    A. X gradient
    B. Y gradient
    C. Z gradient
    D. None of the above

19. During the acquisition of axial images of the body with the frequency direction L/R, phase encoding is performed by which physical gradient?
    A. X gradient
    B. Y gradient
    C. Z gradient
    D. None of the above

20. During the acquisition of sagittal images with the phase direction A/P, frequency encoding is performed by which physical gradient?
    A. X gradient
    B. Y gradient
    C. Z gradient
    D. None of the above

21. During the acquisition of coronal images with the phase direction L/R, frequency encoding is conducted by which physical gradient?
    A. X gradient
    B. Y gradient
    C. Z gradient
    D. None of the above

17.a 18.a 19.b 20.c 21.c

22. During the acquisition of axial images of the body with the phase direction A/P, frequency encoding is performed by which physical gradient?
    A. X gradient
    B. Y gradient
    C. Z gradient
    D. None of the above

23. During the acquisition of axial images of the brain with the phase direction L/R, frequency encoding is performed by which physical gradient?
    A. X gradient
    B. Y gradient
    C. Z gradient
    D. None of the above

24. In MR imaging, slice thickness is determined by which factor(s)?
    A. Magnet field strength
    B. Gradient slope slice select
    C. Transmit bandwidth
    D. Both B and C

25. In MRI, thin slices are achieved by applying a _____ gradient slope or a _____ bandwidth.
    A. Shallow, Broad
    B. Steep, Narrow
    C. Shallow, Narrow
    D. None of the above

26. In MRI, thick slices are achieved by applying a _____ gradient slope or a _____ bandwidth.
    A. Shallow, Broad
    B. Steep, Narrow
    C. Shallow, Narrow
    D. None of the above

22.a 23.b 24.d 25.b 26.a

27. The range of frequencies that is sampled during frequency encoding is known as the _____.
    A. Receive bandwidth
    B. Transmit bandwidth
    C. Gradient slope
    D. None of the above

28. The range of frequencies that is transmitted by the RF pulse is known as the _____.
    A. Receive bandwidth
    B. Transmit bandwidth
    C. Gradient slope
    D. None of the above

29. In MR imaging, the interslice gap is determined by which factor(s)?
    A. Slice selection gradient slope
    B. Slice thickness
    C. External magnetic field strength
    D. Both A and B

30. The gradient that is turned on during the application of the 90 degree excitation pulse and the 180 degree RF pulse is known as _____.
    A. Slice selection gradient
    B. Phase encoding gradient
    C. Frequency encoding gradient
    D. None of the above

31. The gradient that is turned on during signal sampling is known as the _____.
    A. Slice selection gradient
    B. Phase encoding gradient
    C. Frequency encoding gradient
    D. None of the above

27.a 28.b 29.d 30.a 31.c

32. The gradient that is turned on just before the 180 degree rephasing pulse is known as the _____.
    A. Slice selection gradient
    B. Phase encoding gradient
    C. Frequency encoding gradient
    D. None of the above

33. The amplitude of the phase and frequency encoding gradients determines the dimension of what parameter?
    A. FOV
    B. TR
    C. TE
    D. NEX

34. The frequency encoding gradient is also known as the _____ because it is turned on during the sampling of signal.
    A. Refocusing gradient
    B. Spoiler gradient
    C. Readout gradient
    D. Phase encoding gradient

35. The theorem that states that a frequency must be sampled at least twice in order to reproduce it reliably is known as the _____.
    A. Pathagarum theorem
    B. Nyquist theorem
    C. Larmor theorem
    D. Fourier theorem

36. The rate at which signal samples are taken during frequency encoding is known as the _____.
    A. Readout rate
    B. Frequency rate
    C. Sampling rate
    D. None of the above

32.b 33.a 34.c 35.b 36.c

37. During the sampling of signal, the sampling rate is directly proportional to the
_____.
A. Sampling time
B. Receive bandwidth
C. Transmit bandwidth
D. None of the above

38. During the sampling of signal, the sampling time is inversely proportional to
_____.
A. Sampling rate
B. Transmit bandwidth
C. Receive bandwidth
D. Both A and C

39. The spacial location of signal according to its precessional phase is known
as_____.
A. Slice selection
B. Phase encoding
C. Frequency encoding
D. Readout

40. The spacial location of signal according to its precessional frequency is
known as _____.
A. Slice selection
B. Phase encoding
C. Frequency encoding
D. Spoiling

41. The area within the array processor where spatially located information is
stored is known as _____.
A. Interspace
B. Array space
C. Fourier space
D. K space

37.b 38.d 39.b 40.c 41.d

42. The magnitude of the phase shifts between two points within a patient is determined by which factor?
    A. Slope of the frequency encoding gradient
    B. Slope of the phase encoding gradient
    C. Strength of the RF pulse
    D. None of the above

43. The process that uses mathematical conversions to calculate the amplitude of individual frequencies is known as _____.
    A. Fast Fourier transformation
    B. Free induction decay
    C. Larmor equation
    D. None of the above

44. The number of times each signal is sampled with the same value of the phase encoding gradient is known as _____.
    A. Number of signal averages
    B. Number of excitations
    C. Number of signal quotients
    D. All of the above

45. The higher the number of excitations that are acquired the more K space that is filled.
    A. True
    B. False

46. In conventional spin echo sequences, how many phase encoding steps must be selected to fill 128 lines of K space?
    A. 64
    B. 128
    C. 192
    D. 256

42.b 43.a 44.d 45.a 46.b

47. In conventional spin echo sequences, how many phase encoding steps must be selected to fill 256 lines of K space?
    A. 64
    B. 128
    C. 192
    D. 256

48. Which Parameter(s) effect total scan time?
    A. Repetition time
    B. Number of phase encoding steps
    C. Number of excitations
    D. All of the above

49. During a conventional spin echo pulse sequence, each slice is selected, phase encoded, and frequency encoded once per TR.
    A. True
    B. False

50. The horizontal axis of K space represents which axis of the image?
    A. Phase encoding
    B. Frequency encoding
    C. Slice selection
    D. None of the above

51. The vertical axis of K space represents which axis of the image?
    A. Phase encoding
    B. Frequency encoding
    C. Slice selection
    D. None of the above

52. The area of K space filled with the shallowest phase encoding slopes is known as _____.
    A. Central lines
    B. Outer lines
    C. Negative lines only
    D. None of the above

47.d 48.d 49.a 50.a 51.b 52.a

53. The area of K space that is filled with the steepest phase encoding gradient slopes is known as _____.
    A. Central lines
    B. Outer lines
    C. Positive lines only
    D. None of the above

54. Image data along both the phase and frequency axis with the highest signal amplitude is stored in which area of K space?
    A. Central lines
    B. Outer lines
    C. Positive lines only
    D. None of the above

55. Image data along both the phase and frequency axis with the lowest signal amplitude is stored in which area of the K space?
    A. Central lines
    B. Outer lines
    C. Positive lines only
    D. None of the above

56. When the phase encoding gradient is activated, steep slopes produce what type of signal amplitude?
    A. High
    B. Low
    C. Medium
    D. None of the above

57. When the phase encoding gradient is activated, shallow slopes produce what type of signal amplitude?
    A. High
    B. Low
    C. Medium
    D. None of the above

53.b 54.a 55.b 56.b 57.a

58. When the phase encoding gradient is activated, medium slopes produce what type of signal amplitudes?
    A. High
    B. Low
    C. Medium
    D. None of the above

59. When the amplitude of the phase encoding gradient increases, the amount of phase shift along the gradient _____.
    A. Increases
    B. Decreases
    C. Stays the same
    D. None of the above

60. When the phase encoding gradient is activated, steep slopes produce data with what type of spatial resolution?
    A. High
    B. Low
    C. Medium
    D. None of the above

61. Image data with high spatial resolution is stored in which area of K space?
    A. Outer lines
    B. Central lines
    C. Negative lines only
    D. Positive lines only

62. Image data with low spatial resolution is stored in which area of K space?
    A. Outer lines
    B. Central lines
    C. Negative lines only
    D. Positive lines only

58.c 59.a 60.a 61.a 62.b

63. The process of filling K space by sampling only half of the echo and interpolating the rest is known as _____.
    A. Fractional echo
    B. Gradient echo
    C. Partial echo
    D. Both A and C

64. The process of filling only a percentage of K space with acquired data and filling the rest with zeros is known as _____.
    A. Partial saturation
    B. Partial averaging
    C. Partial voluming
    D. Partial echo

65. Which method of image acquisition acquires all of the data from one slice before acquiring data from the next slice?
    A. Sequential
    B. 2D volumetric
    C. 3D volumetric
    D. None of the above

66. Which method of image acquisition fills one line of K space for each slice in the sequence before it moves to the second line of K space?
    A. Sequential
    B. 2D volumetric
    C. 3D volumetric
    D. None of the above

67. Which method of image acquisition acquires data from an entire volume of tissue, then uses a method called slice encoding to separate the images?
    A. Sequential
    B. 2D volumetric
    C. 3D volumetric

63.d 64.b 65.a 66.b 67.c

HALF-FOURIER

OR FRACTIONAL AVERAGING

PARTIAL FOURIER

68. The thickness of an MRI image can be changed by which of the following methods?
    A. Altering the gradient slope
    B. Changing the number of excitations
    C. Altering the RF bandwidth
    D. Both A and C

69. The term used to describe a volume element is known as _____.
    A. Pixel
    B. Pixie
    C. Voxel
    D. Picture element

70. The number of picture elements used to make up an image is known as _____.
    A. Contrast
    B. Matrix
    C. Signal to noise
    D. None of the above

71. The ability to distinguish one structure from another on an image is known as _____.
    A. Spatial resolution
    B. Contrast to noise
    C. Signal to noise
    D. None of the above

72. The term used to describe a picture element is known as a _____.
    A. Image element
    B. Pixel
    C. Voxel
    D. Volume element

68.d 69.c 70.b 71.a 72.b

73. The size of the area being displayed on an MR image is known as _____.
    A. Field of view
    B. Voxel size
    C. Pixel size
    D. None of the above

74. The depth of a volume element is determined by what parameter?
    A. Matrix
    B. NEX
    C. Repetition time
    D. Slice thickness

75. The height and width of a picture element is determined by what parameter(s)?
    A. Size of the FOV
    B. Number of phase encoding steps
    C. Number of frequency encoding steps
    D. All of the above

76. A volume element that has the same height, width, and depth is known as _____.
    A. Rectangular
    B. Isotropic
    C. Triangular
    D. Anisotropic

77. A voxel that is unequal in height, width, and depth is known as _____.
    A. Isotropic
    B. Triangular
    C. Square
    D. Anisotropic

73.a 74.d 75.d 76.b 77.d

78. Three characteristics commonly used to define the quality of an MRI image are _____.
   A. Contrast, Resolution, Matrix
   B. Resolution, Contrast, Signal to noise
   C. Signal to noise, Excitations, Contrast
   D. Resolution, Matrix, Signal to noise

79. The difference in brightness between two regions of an image is known as _____.
   A. Signal to noise
   B. Image contrast
   C. Spacial resolution
   D. None of the above

80. Bright pixels on an MRI image represent what type of signal?
   A. Low
   B. High
   C. Weak
   D. None of the above

81. The clarity with which different areas of an image are distinguished is known as _____.
   A. Image contrast
   B. Signal to noise
   C. Spacial resolution
   D. None of the above

82. The proportion of signal actually used to construct an image relative to the amount of background noise is known as _____.
   A. Spacial resolution
   B. Signal to noise ratio
   C. Image contrast
   D. None of the above

78.b 79.b 80.b 81.c 82.b

83. An image with a grainy appearance usually represents an image with _____.
    A. High resolution
    B. Low signal to noise
    C. High signal to noise
    D. Low resolution

84. Noise that degrades image quality in a specific location within an MRI image is known as _____.
    A. Inherent noise interference
    B. Random noise interference
    C. Discrete noise interference
    D. None of the above

85. Noise that generally degrades overall quality of an MRI image is known as_____.
    A. Inherent noise interference
    B. Random noise interference
    C. Discrete noise interference
    D. None of the above

86. Which of the following is a parameter that directly affects signal to noise ratio?
    A. Voxel size
    B. Number of excitations
    C. Repetition time
    D. All of the above

87. The term *"Trade-off parameters"* is used to describe parameters that affect each other inversely.
    A. True
    B. False

83.b 84.c 85.b 86.d 87.a

88. When magnetic field strength increases, signal to noise ratio_____.
    A. Increases
    B. Decreases
    C. Stays the same

89. When voxel size decreases, signal to noise ratio_____.
    A. Increases
    B. Decreases
    C. Stays the same

90. When pixel size increases, signal to noise ratio_____.
    A. Increases
    B. Decreases
    C. Stays the same

91. When bandwidth is increased, signal to noise ratio_____.
    A. Increases
    B. Decreases
    C. Stays the same

92. When repetition time is increased, signal to noise ratio _____.
    A. Increases
    B. Decreases
    C. Stays the same

93. When echo time is increased, signal to noise ratio _____.
    A. Increases
    B. Decreases
    C. Stays the same

88.a 89.b 90.a 91.b 92.a 93.b

94. When field of view decreases, spacial resolution_____.
     A. Increases
     B. Decreases
     C. Stays the same

95. When field of view is increased, signal to noise ratio_____.
     A. Increases
     B. Decreases
     C. Stays the same

96. When the number of excitations is increased, spacial resolution_____.
     A. Increases
     B. Decreases
     C. Stays the same

97. When image matrix is increased, spacial resolution_____.
     A. Increases
     B. Decreases
     C. Stays the same

98. When slice thickness is increased, signal to noise ratio_____.
     A. Increases
     B. Decreases
     C. Stays the same

99. When slice spacing increases, signal to noise ratio_____.
     A. Increases
     B. Decreases
     C. Stays the same

94.a 95.a 96.c 97.a 98.a 99.a

100. When image matrix is decreased, spacial resolution _____.
    A. Increases
    B. Decreases
    C. Stays the same

101. When TE is decreased, the spacial resolution_____.
    A. Increases
    B. Decreases
    C. Stays the same

102. When TR is increased, acquisition time _____.
    A. Increases
    B. Decreases
    C. Stays the same

103. When the number of excitations is decreased, acquisition time_____.
    A. Increases
    B. Decreases
    C. Stays the same

104. When image matrix increases, acquisition time _____.
    A. Increases
    B. Decreases
    C. Stays the same

105. With the parameters given, which protocol gives the highest signal to noise ratio?
    A. Long TR/Short TE/ High matrix
    B. Short TR/Long TE/ Low matrix
    C. Long TR/LongTE/High matrix
    D. Long TR/Short TE/Low matrix

100.b 101.c 102.a 103.b 104.a 105.d

106. With the parameters given, which protocol gives the highest spacial resolution?
   A. Thick slice/Large FOV/High matrix
   B. Thin slice/Large FOV/High matrix
   C. Thin slice/Small FOV/Low matrix
   D. Thin slice/Small FOV/High matrix

107. With the parameters given, which protocol has the longest acquisition time?
   A. Long TR/Low NEX/Low matrix
   B. Short TR/High NEX/Low matrix
   C. Short TR/Low NEX/High matrix
   D. Long TR/High NEX/High matrix

108. With the parameters given, which protocol gives the highest signal to noise ratio?
   A. Thick slice/Low TE/Large FOV
   B. Thin slice/High TE/Small FOV
   C. Thick slice/High TE/Small FOV
   D. Thin slice/Low TE/Small FOV

109. As bandwidth increases, sampling time _____.
   A. Increases
   B. Decreases
   C. Stays the same

110. As bandwidth decreases, sampling time _____.
   A. Increases
   B. Decreases
   C. Stays the same

106.d 107.d 108.a 109.b 110.a
X B

60

111. Which of the following *logical* gradients is known as the frequency encoding gradient?
    A. X gradient
    B. Y gradient
    C. Z gradient

112. Which of the following *logical* gradients is known as the phase encoding gradient?
    A. X gradient
    B. Y gradient
    C. Z gradient

113. Which of the following *logical* gradients is known as the slice selection gradient?
    A. X gradient
    B. Y gradient
    C. Z gradient

114. In plane pixel size can be determined by which of the following methods?
    A. Dividing the FOV by the number phase and frequency steps
    B. Dividing the NEX by the FOV
    C. Dividing the TR by the NEX
    D. Dividing the TR by the slice thickness

115. Which of the following is the formula for determining scan time for a 3D FT pulse sequence?
    A. TR x NEX x phase steps x number of slices
    B. TR x NEX x phase steps
    C. NEX x TR x number of slices
    D. TR x phase steps x number of slices

111.a 112.b 113.c 114.a 115.a

Exercise 4-1

Draw an arrow showing the effects that each parameter has on SNR,
Spacial Resolution, and Scan Time.

Increase ↑ Decrease ↓	Signal to Noise Ratio	Spacial Resolution	Scan Time
↑ TR			
↑ TE			
↓ NEX			
↓ Matrix			
↑ Slice Thickness			
↑ FOV			
↓ Slice Gap			

SECTION 5

Pulse Sequences

Spin Echo Pulse Sequences
Gradient Echo Pulse Sequences

1. The type of pulse sequence that uses only 90 degree RF pulses is known as _____.
   A. Partial saturation pulse sequence   p 66 (Bushong)
   B. Gradient echo pulse sequence
   C. Saturation recovery pulse sequence
   D. Both A and B

2. A spin echo pulse sequence is characterized by which of the following?
   A. A 180 degree excitation pulse followed by a 90 degree rephasing pulse
   B. A 90 degree excitation pulse followed by a 180 degree rephasing pulse
   C. A 90 degree excitation pulse followed by a 90 degree rephasing pulse
   D. None of the above

3. Which of the following is the pulse sequence that is used most commonly?
   A. Inversion recovery
   B. Gradient echo
   C. Spin echo
   D. Echo planar

4. Which of the following is an advantage of using a spin echo pulse sequence?
   A. High signal to noise ratio
   B. Decreased resolution
   C. Long scan times
   D. None of the above

5. In conventional spin echo pulse sequences, how many phase encoding steps are achieved per TR?
   A. 1
   B. 128
   C. 192
   D. 256

1.d 2.b 3.c 4.a 5.a

p66 Bush.

A,B & C

6. In conventional spin echo pulse sequences, how many lines of K space are filled per TR?
   - A. 1
   - B. 2
   - C. 4
   - D. 6

7. The spin echo pulse sequence that performs more than one phase encoding step per TR is known as _____.
   - A. Conventional spin echo
   - B. Fast spin echo
   - C. RARE
   - D. Both B and C

8. The pulse sequence that performs a series of 180 degree rephasing pulses and echos is known as _____.
   - A. Echo planar
   - B. Inversion recovery
   - C. Fast spin echo
   - D. Conventional spin echo

9. The series of 180 degree rephasing pulses in a fast spin echo pulse sequence is known as _____.
   - A. Echo train
   - B. Inversion train
   - C. Echo plane
   - D. None of the above

10. The number of 180 degree rephasing pulses performed in a fast spin echo pulse sequence is known as its _____.
   - A. Turbo factor
   - B. Inversion factor
   - C. Echo train length
   - D. Both A and C

6.a 7.d 8.c 9.a 10.d

11. In a RARE pulse sequence, the multiple number of echo times that create image weighting are averaged together to produce what is known as the _____.
    A. Effective TR
    B. Effective TI
    C. Effective TE
    D. None of the above

12. Which of the following is an advantage of a fast spin echo pulse sequence?
    A. Reduced scan times
    B. Improved quality
    C. Increased T2 weighting
    D. All of the above

13. Which of the following is a disadvantage of fast spin echo pulse sequences?
    A. Increased effects of flow motion
    B. Bright fat on T2 weighted images
    C. Increased resolution
    D. Both A and B

14. The type of spin echo pulse sequence that begins with a 180 degree inversion RF pulse and is followed by a 90 degree excitation pulse is known as _____.
    A Echo planar
    B. Gradient echo
    C. Inversion recovery
    D. Gradient reversal

15. During an inversion recovery pulse sequence, the time between the 180 degree inversion pulse and the 90 degree excitation pulse is known as _____.
    A. Echo time
    B. Repetition time
    C. Inversion time
    D. Reversion time

11.c 12.d 13.d 14.c 15.c

16. The inversion recovery pulse sequence that is used to suppress fat in a T1 weighted image is known as _____.
    A. FLAIR
    B. STIR
    C. SSFP
    D. FLASH

17. The inversion recovery pulse sequence that is used to suppress CSF in proton density and T2 weighted images is known as _____.
    A. FLAIR
    B. STIR
    C. SSFP
    D. FISP

18. The type of pulse sequence that uses a gradient instead of a 180 degree RF pulse to rephase dephasing nuclei is known as _____.
    A. Spin echo
    B. Inversion recovery
    C. Fast spin echo
    D. Gradient echo

19. In a gradient echo pulse sequence, which gradient is used to dephase and rephase nuclei? See p. 114 MRIP
    A. Slice select gradient
    B. Phase encoding gradient
    C. Frequency encoding gradient
    D. None of the above

20. In a gradient echo pulse sequence, which parameter directly affects image weighting?
    A. NEX
    B. Field of view
    C. Flip angle
    D. Matrix

16.b 17.a 18.d 19.c 20.c

21. The condition that occurs in a gradient echo pulse sequence when the TR is shorter than the T1 and T2 relaxation times of tissue is known as _____.
    A. Chemical shift
    B. Steady state
    C. Frequency shift
    D. Phase shift

22. In a gradient echo pulse sequence, transverse magnetization that is leftover from a previous excitation pulse is known as _____.
    A. Residual transverse magnetization
    B. Magnetization transfer
    C. Chemical misregistration
    D. None of the above

23. Gradient echo pulse sequences that preserve left over transverse magnetization are said to be _____.
    A. Incoherent
    B. Coherent
    C. Consistent
    D. Inconsistent

24. Gradient echo pulse sequences that eliminate leftover transverse magnetization are said to be _____.
    A. Incoherent
    B. Coherent
    C. Consistent
    D. Inconsistent

25. In a gradient echo pulse sequence, the process of reversing the slope of the phase encoding gradient after readout to preserve residual transverse magnetization is known as _____.
    A. Warping
    B. Spoiling
    C. Rewinding
    D. None of the above

21.b 22.a 23.b 24.a 25.c

26. In a gradient echo pulse sequence, the process of eliminating residual transverse magnetization is known as _____.
    A. Warping
    B. Spoiling
    C. Rewinding
    D. None of the above

27. Which of the following is a method of eliminating residual transverse magnetization?
    A. Digital RF spoiling
    B. Gradient rewinding
    C. Gradient spoiling
    D. Both A and C

28. In a gradient echo pulse sequence, the use of an RF pulse to eliminate residual transverse magnetization is known as _____.
    A. Digital RF spoiling
    B. Frequency spoiling
    C. Gradient spoiling
    D. None of the above

29. In a gradient echo pulse sequence, the use of a gradient to eliminate residual transverse magnetization is known as _____.
    A. Digital RF spoiling
    B. Frequency spoiling
    C. Gradient spoiling
    D. None of the above

30. Gradient echo pulse sequences that have incoherent residual transverse magnetization are primarily used to create what type of image weighting?
    A. T1 weighting
    B. T2 weighting
    C. Proton density weighting
    D. Both A and C

26.b 27.d 28.a 29.c 30.d

31. Gradient echo pulse sequences that have coherent residual transverse magnetization produce what type of image weighting?
    A. T1 weighting
    B. T2* weighting
    C. Proton density weighting
    D. Both A and C

32. Which of the following is an advantage of gradient echo pulse sequences?
    A. Decreased scan time
    B. Increased sensitivity to flow
    C. Volume acquisitions possible
    D. All of the above

33. Which of the following is a disadvantage of a gradient echo pulse sequence?
    A. Decreased signal to noise ratio
    B. Increased sensitivity to magnetic susceptibility artifacts
    C. Increased gradient noise
    D. All of the above

34. The gradient echo pulse sequence that produces true T2 image weighting is known as _____.
    A. SSFP
    B. T2 FFE
    C. PSIF
    D. All of the above

35. The gradient echo pulse sequence that is characterized by an echo time that is longer than its repetition time is known as _____.
    A. Echo planar
    B. Steady state free precession
    C. Spin echo
    D. Fast spin echo

See p. 124 MR≠P

31.b 32.d 33.d 34.d 35.b

36. The type of pulse sequence that fills all lines of K space per TR
    is known as _____.
    A. Fast spin echo
    B. Steady state free precession
    C. Echo planar
    D. Spin echo

37. In an echo planar pulse sequence, using a long TE produces what type of
    weighting?
    A. T1 weighting
    B. T2 weighting
    C. Proton density weighting
    D. None of the above

38. In an echo planar pulse sequence, pre-inverting tissue with a 180 degree RF
    pulse before excitation produces what type of image weighting?
    A. T1 weighting
    B. T2 weighting
    C. Proton density weighting
    D. None of the above

39. In an echo planar pulse sequence, proton density weighting can be produced
    by which of the following techniques?
    A. Applying a 180 degree RF pulse to pre-invert tissue before excitation
    B. Using a short TE
    C. Using a long TE
    D. Using a 180 degree rephasing pulse

36.c 37.b 38.a 39.b

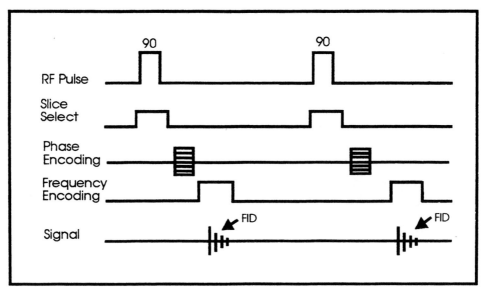

Figure 5-1

40. Figure 5-1 is a diagram showing what type of pulse sequence?
    A. Partial saturation
    B. Spin echo
    C. Inversion recovery
    D. Gradient echo

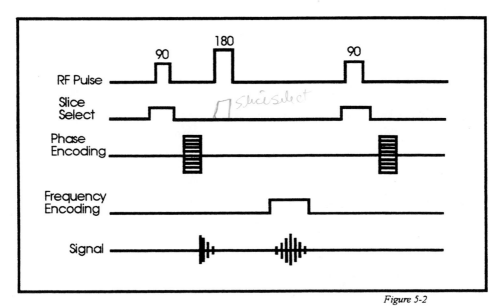

Figure 5-2

40.a

41. Figure 5-2 is a diagram showing what type of pulse sequence?
    A. Partial saturation
    B. Spin echo
    C. Inversion recovery
    D. Gradient echo

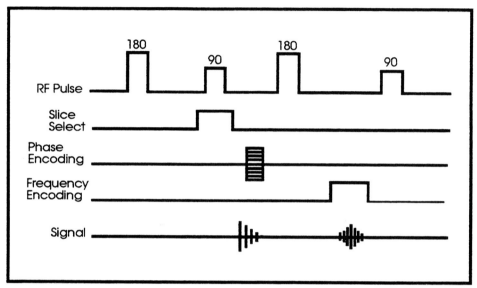

Figure 5-3

42. Figure 5-3 is a diagram showing what type of pulse sequence?
    A. Partial saturation
    B. Spin echo
    C. Inversion recovery
    D. Gradient echo

41.b 42.c

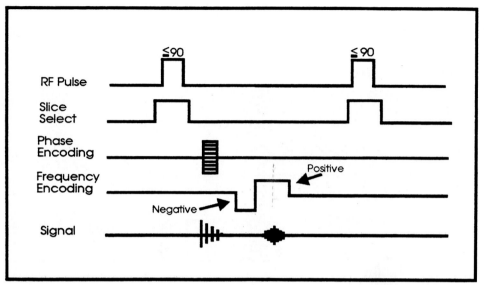

Figure 5-4

43. Figure 5-4 is a diagram showing what type of pulse sequence?
    A. Partial saturation
    B. Spin echo
    C. Inversion recovery
    D. Gradient Echo

44. Which of the following methods can reduce blurring in a fast spin echo pulse sequence?
    A. Reduce echo train length
    B. Reduce resolution
    C. Reduce TR
    D. Reduce effective TE

45. During a fast spin echo pulse sequence, which lines of k space are filled by the gradients performed closest to the effective TE?
    A. Central lines
    B. Outer lines
    C. Negative lines only
    D. Positive lines only

43.d 44.a 45.a

General Electric Pulse Sequences

MEMP	Multi Echo Multi Planar
VEMP	Variable Echo Multi Planar
FSE	Fast Spin Echo
GRASS	Gradient Recalled Acquisition at a Steady State
SPGR	Spoiled Gradient Recalled Acquisition at a Steady State
MPGR	Multi Planar Gradient Recalled Acquisition at a Steady State
SSFP	Steady State Free Precession
MPIR	Multi Planar Inversion Recovery
STIR	Short TI Inversion Recovery

Philips Pulse Sequences

SE	Spin Echo
TSE	Turbo Spin Echo
FFE	Fast Field Echo
T1FFE	T1 Fast Field Echo
T2FFE	T2 Fast Field Echo
IR	Inversion Recovery
SPIR	Spectrally Selective Inversion Recovery

Picker Pulse Sequences

SE	Spin Echo
FSE	Fast Spin Echo
FAST	Fourier Acquired Steady State Technique
RF Spoiled Fast	RF Spoiled Fourier Acquired Steady State Technique
CE Fast	Contrast Enhanced Fourier Acquired Steady State Technique
IR	Inversion Recovery
STIR	Short TI Inversion Recovery

Siemens Pulse Sequences

SE	Spin Echo
TSE	Turbo Spin Echo
FISP	Fast Imaging with Steady Precession
FLASH	Fast Low Angle Shot
PSIF	Mirrored Fast Imaging with Steady Precession
IR	Inversion Recovery
STIR	Short TI Inversion Recovery

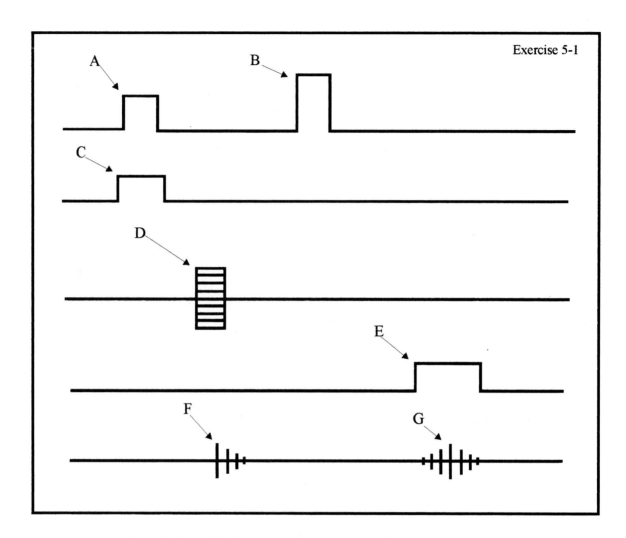

Place the letter in the space that corresponds to the proper part of the pulse sequence.

_____ Spin Echo Signal   _____ Readout Gradient

_____ Phase Encoding Gradient   _____ Slice Select Gradient

_____ 180° Radio Frequency Pulse _____ 90° Radio Frequency Pulse

_____ FID Signal

SECTION 6

Artifacts and Corrections

Phase Mismapping
Aliasing
Chemical Shift
Chemical Misregistration
Gibbs
Magnetic Susceptibility
Zipper
Cross Excitation
Cross Talk
Shading

1. An image artifact caused by anatomical motion along a gradient is known as what type of artifact?
    A. Ringing
    B. Aliasing
    C. Volume averaging
    D. Phase mismapping

2. Another name for phase mismapping artifact is _____.
    A. Ringing
    B. Aliasing
    C. Ghosting
    D. Truncation

3. An example of phase mismapping artifact is _____.
    A. Cardiac motion
    B. Flow motion
    C. Respiratory motion
    D. All of the above

4. An example of aperiodic motion is _____.
    A. Cardiac motion
    B. Flow motion
    C. Respiratory motion
    D. Peristalsis motion

5. Ghosting artifact on an MR image caused by the heart can be decreased by which of the following methods?
    A. Decreasing bandwidth
    B. Peripheral compensation
    C. Cardiac gating
    D. Respiratory compensation

1.d 2.c 3.d 4.d 5.c

6. Motion artifact on an MR image caused by flowing blood or CSF can be decreased by which of the following methods?
   A. Respiratory compensation
   B. Patient education
   C. Gradient moment nulling
   D. Respiratory gating

7. Peripheral gating is a technique used to decrease what type of motion artifact?
   A. CSF pulsation motion
   B. Cardiac motion
   C. Swallowing
   D. Respiratory motion

8. A saturation pulse is a technique used to reduce what type of motion artifact?
   A. Blood flow motion
   B. Respiratory motion
   C. Swallowing motion
   D. All of the above

9. Phase mismapping artifact always occurs in which direction of the MR image?
   A. Frequency direction
   B. Phase direction
   C. Slice selection direction
   D. Readout direction

10. Phase mismapping artifact caused by respiratory motion can be decreased by which method?
    A. Presaturation pulse
    B. Swapping phase and frequency direction
    C. Respiratory compensation
    D. All of the above

6.c 7.a 8.d 9.b 10.d

11. Gradient moment nulling is most effective in reducing flow related motion in which type of flow?
    A. Slow flow
    B. Fast flow
    C. Inplane flow
    D. Both A and C

12. The artifact that is produced when anatomy that is outside the FOV is mapped within the FOV is known as _____.
    A. Phase mismapping
    B. Aliasing
    C. Partial volume averaging
    D. Magnetic susceptibility

13. Another name for aliasing artifact is _____.
    A. Foldover artifact
    B. Ringing artifact
    C. Wraparound artifact
    D. Both A and C

14. Wraparound artifact occurs in which direction of an MR image?
    A. Phase direction
    B. Frequency direction
    C. Slice selection direction
    D. Both A and B

15. Wraparound artifact caused by undersampling of frequencies in the readout direction is known as _____.
    A. Phase wrap
    B. Frequency wrap
    C. Gibbs wrap
    D. Truncation

11.d 12.b 13. d 14.d 15.b

16. Foldover artifact caused by undersampling of signal in the phase encoding direction is known as _____.
    A. Phase wrap
    B. Frequency wrap
    C. Gibbs wrap
    D. None of the above

17. Aliasing artifact in the frequency direction can be corrected by which of the following methods?
    A. Decreasing the FOV
    B. Increasing the matrix
    C. Filtering the frequencies outside the FOV in the phase direction
    D. Filtering the frequencies outside the FOV in the frequency direction

18. Foldover artifact in the phase direction can be corrected by which of the following methods?
    A. Oversampling signal outside the FOV
    B. Increasing the FOV
    C. Using saturation pulses outside the FOV
    D. All of the above

19. The precessional frequency of hydrogen is influenced by its chemical environment.
    A. True
    B. False

20. In fat, the hydrogen atom is bound with what other type of atom?
    A. Oxygen
    B. Nitrogen
    C. Helium
    D. Carbon

16.a 17.d 18.d 19.a 20.d

21. In water, the hydrogen atom is bound with what other type of atom?
    A. Oxygen
    B. Nitrogen
    C. Helium
    D. Carbon

22. The artifact that is caused due to the difference in precessional frequencies between fat and water is called _____.
    A. Magnetic susceptibility
    B. Chemical shift
    C. Truncation
    D. Aliasing

23. In a 1.5 tesla magnet, the difference in the precessional frequency between fat and water is _____.
    A. 250 MHz
    B. 210 MHz
    C. 220 watts
    D. 220 Hz

24. In a 1.0 tesla magnet, the difference in the precessional frequency between fat and water is _____.
    A. 130 MHz
    B. 147 Hz
    C. 200 Hz
    D. 220 Hz

25. Chemical shift artifact occurs in which direction of the MR image?
    A. Phase encoding direction
    B. Frequency encoding direction
    C. Slice selection direction
    D. None of the above

21.a 22.b 23.d 24.b 25.b

26. In an MR image, the degree of chemical shift artifact depends upon which parameter?
    A. Receive bandwidth
    B. Size of the FOV
    C. Magnetic field strength
    D. All of the above

27. Chemical shift artifact can be minimized by which of the following methods?
    A. Minimizing the FOV
    B. Increasing the receive bandwidth
    C. Utilizing chemical saturation
    D. All of the above

28. The artifact that is caused by the phase differences between fat and water is known as _____.
    A. Chemical shift
    B. Phase wrap
    C. Chemical misregistration
    D. Ringing

29. Chemical misregistration artifact most commonly occurs in which direction of the MR image?
    A. Phase encoding direction
    B. Frequency encoding direction
    C. Slice selection direction
    D. None of the above

30. Chemical misregistration artifact is most likely to affect which type of pulse sequence?
    A. Spin echo pulse sequences
    B. Inversion recovery pulse sequences
    C. Gradient echo pulse sequences
    D. None of the above

26.d 27.d 28.c 29.a 30.c

31. Which imaging parameter affects the amount of chemical misregistration that will be seen on an image?
    A. TR
    B. TI
    C. TE
    D. NEX

32. At 1.5 tesla, to reduce chemical misregistration artifact, the TE should be a multiple of what time?
    A. 3.1 ms
    B. 4.2 ms
    C. 6.6 ms
    D. 7.3 ms

33. At .5 tesla, to reduce chemical misregistration artifact, the TE should be a multiple of what time?
    A. 3.1 ms
    B. 4.2 ms
    C. 6.6 ms
    D. 7.0 ms

34. The time that both fat and water are in phase with each other is known as _____.
    A. Periodicity
    B. Repetition time
    C. Inversion time
    D. None of the above

35. Another name for truncation artifact is _____.
    A. Foldover artifact
    B. Gibbs artifact
    C. Ringing artifact
    D. Both B and C

31.c 32.b 33.d 34.a 35.d

36. The artifact that appears as a low intensity band in areas of high intensity due to undersampling is known as _____.
    A. Gibbs artifact
    B. Truncation artifact
    C. Ringing artifact
    D. All of the above

37. Gibbs artifact can be decreased by _____ the number of phase encoding steps.
    A. Increasing
    B. Decreasing

38. Truncation artifact occurs in which direction of the MRI image?
    A. Phase encoding direction
    B. Frequency encoding direction
    C. Slice selection direction
    D. None of the above

39. Metal in the patient, in the area that is being scanned, will most likely create what type of artifact?
    A. Foldover artifact
    B. Chemical shift artifact
    C. Truncation artifact
    D. Magnetic susceptability

40. Magnetic susceptibility artifact is most prominent in what type of pulse sequence?
    A. Spin echo
    B. Inversion recovery
    C. Gradient echo
    D. None of the above

36.d 37.a 38.a 39.d 40.c

41. Magnetic susceptibility artifact can be used to help diagnose what pathology?
    A. Torn meniscus
    B. Herniated nucleus pulposis
    C. Pituitary adenoma
    D. Hemorrhage

42. An artifact that is caused by an external radio frequency leak is known as _____.
    A. Shading artifact
    B. Zipper artifact
    C. Starring artifact
    D. Herringbone

43. In clinical MRI, what method is used to prevent external radio frequency from affecting the MRI image?
    A. Copper shielded room
    B. Iron shielded magnet
    C. Passive shimming
    D. None of the above

44. The artifact that is produced by overlapping radio frequency pulses in adjacent slices is known as _____.
    A. Cross excitation artifact
    B. Aliasing artifact
    C. Truncation artifact
    D. Phase mismapping artifact

45. The artifact produced by the transfer of spin lattice energy from one slice to its adjacent slice is known as _____.
    A. Wraparound artifact
    B. Ringing artifact
    C. Cross talk artifact
    D. Magnetic susceptibility

41.d 42.b 43.a 44.a 45.c

46. Cross excitation artifact can be eliminated by which of the following methods?
    A. Increasing interslice gap
    B. Using a sinc RF pulse
    C. Interleaving
    D. All of the above

47. The technique used to eliminate cross excitation artifact that acquires data in two separate acquisitions from alternating slices is known as _____.
    A. Aliasing
    B. Interleaving
    C. Spin warping
    D. None of the above

48. To decrease the chances of cross excitation there should be at least what percentage of interslice gap?
    A. 10 %
    B. 15 %
    C. 30 %
    D. 50 %

49. Cross excitation artifact is less likely to occur with which pulse sequence?
    A. Spin echo, 90 degree flip angle, 10% interslice gap
    B. Spin echo, 90 degree flip angle, 50% interslice gap
    C. Gradient echo, 15 degree flip angle, 30% interslice gap
    D. Dual echo, 90 degree flip angle, 25% interslice gap

50. The artifact that is produced when many structures with different signal intensities are averaged together within a pixel is known as _____.
    A. Cross talk artifact
    B. Truncation artifact
    C. Partial volume averaging
    D. Aliasing artifact

46.d 47.b 48.c 49.c 50.c

51. Volume averaging artifact can be reduced by which of the following methods?
    A. Increasing slice thickness
    B. Decreasing slice thickness
    C. Increasing NEX
    D. Decreasing NEX

52. The artifact that is characterized by a loss of signal intensity in one area of an image is known as _____.
    A. Aliasing artifact
    B. Ringing artifact
    C. Shading artifact
    D. None of the above

53. Shading artifact can be caused by what factor(s)?
    A. Inhomogeneity of the external magnetic field
    B. Undersampling of phase encoding steps
    C. Inhomogeneity of the RF pulse
    D. Both A and C

54. Data loss due to gradient instability, excessive noise, or tuning errors can cause an artifact with what type of appearance?
    A. Zippering
    B. Shading
    C. Staring
    D. Herringbone

55. An artifact caused by faulty receiver attenuation settings during prescan is known as _____.
    A. Herringbone
    B. Shading
    C. Data clipping
    D. Aliasing

51.b 52.c 53.d 54.d 55.c

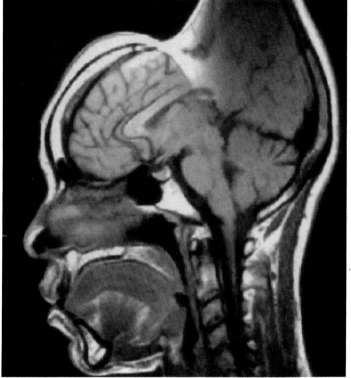

Figure 6-1

56. Figure 6 - 1 displays an example of what type of artifact?
    A. Aliasing
    B. Truncation
    C. Foldover
    D. Magnetic Susceptibility

56.d

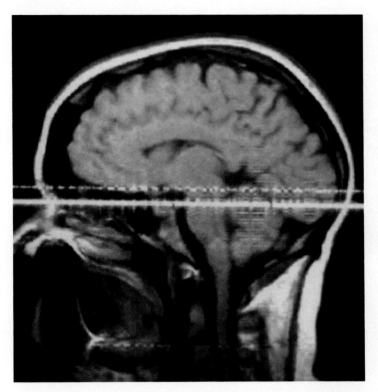

Figure 6-2

57. Figure 6-2 displays an example of what type of artifact?
     A. Magnetic Susceptibility
     B. Phase wrap
     C. RF zipper
     D. Both A and C

57.d

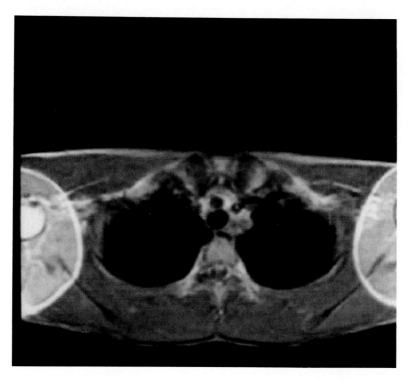

Figure 6-3

58. Figure 6-3 displays an example of what type of artifact?
    A. Ringing
    B. Phase wrap
    C. Chemical shift
    D. Cross talk

58.b

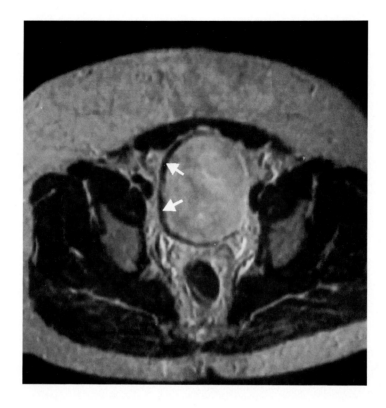

Figure 6-4

59. Figure 6-4 displays an example of what type of artifact?
    A. Phase mismapping
    B. Aliasing
    C. Chemical shift
    D. Cross excitation

59.c

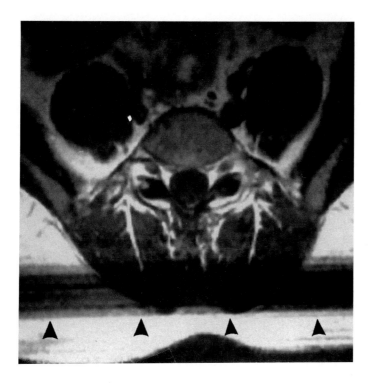

Figure 6-5

60. Figure 6-5 displays an example of what type of artifact?
   A. Truncation
   B. Aliasing
   C. Cross excitation
   D. Chemical shift

60.c

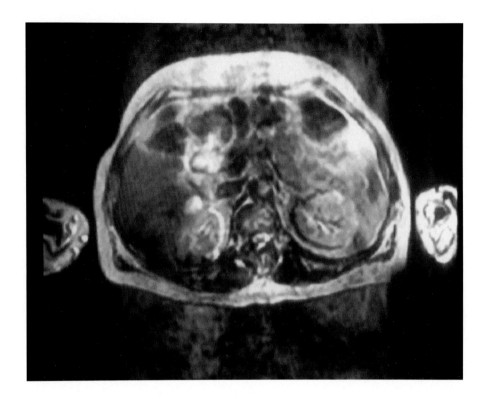

Figure 6-6

61. Figure 6-6 displays an example of what type of artifact?
    A. Aliasing
    B. Truncation
    C. Chemical shift
    D. Phase mismapping

61.d

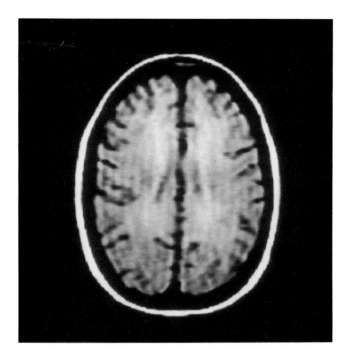

Figure 6-7

62. Figure 6-7 displays an example of what type of artifact?
    A. Aliasing
    B. Truncation
    C. Chemical shift
    D. Phase mismapping

62.b

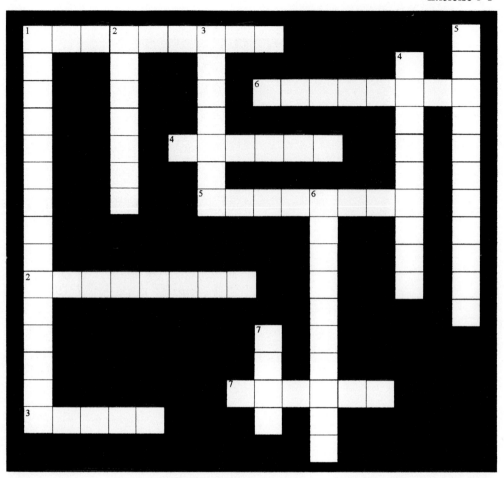

ACROSS

1. Another name for Aliasing artifact.

2. Another name for Foldover artifact.

3. Another name for Truncation artifact.

4. External RF artifact.

5. Respiratory motion artifact.

6. Another name for Phase Wrap artifact.

7. An artifact caused by an uncooperative patient.

DOWN

1. Another name for Ghosting artifact.

2. Artifact caused by inhomogeneity of the external magnetic field.

3. Another name for Gibbs artifact.

4. Volume _____.

5. Artifact named after a fish skeleton.

6. Another name for Ringing artifact.

7. Type of artifact caused by vascular structures.

SECTION 7

1. Blood flow that has consistent velocities within a vessel is known as what type of flow?
    A. Turbulent flow
    B. Laminar flow
    C. Vortex flow
    D. Stagnant flow

2. Blood flow that has randomly different velocities is known as what type of flow?
    A. Turbulent flow
    B. Laminar flow
    C. Vortex flow
    D. Stagnant flow

3. Blood flow that has high velocities in the center of the vessel but spirals near walls of a vessel due to a stricture is known as what type of flow?
    A. Turbulent flow
    B. Laminar flow
    C. Vortex flow
    D. Stagnant flow

4. Blood flow that slows to a point of immobility is known as what type of flow?
    A. Turbulent flow
    B. Laminar flow
    C. Vortex flow
    D. Stagnant flow

5. Blood flow velocity is measured in what type of unit?
    A. Gauss/sec
    B. mm./sec
    C. cm./sec
    D. inches/sec

```
1.b  2.a  3.c  4.d  5.c
```

6. Which of the following is the formula that is used to calculate blood flow velocity?
   A. Velocity = Flow volume / Vessel area
   B. Velocity = Vessel area / Flow volume
   C. Velocity = Flow volume + vessel area
   D. Velocity = Vessel area - Flow volume

7. Blood flow velocity is greatest near which area of the vessel?
   A. Vessel walls
   B. Vessel center
   C. None of the above

8. Blood flow velocity at a given point is dependent upon which factor?
   A. Patient sex
   B. Phase of patient's cardiac cycle
   C. Patient's weight
   D. None of the above

9. During *peak systolic* phase of the cardiac cycle, blood flow velocities are dependent upon what factor(s)?
   A. Patient age
   B. Cardiac output
   C. Anatomical site
   D. All of the above

10. Which of the following vessels has the highest peak velocity?
    A. Ascending aorta
    B. Distal aorta
    C. Proximal carotids
    D. Basilar artery

6.a 7.b 8.b 9.d 10.a

11. Which of the following vessels has the slowest peak velocity?
     A. Ascending aorta
     B. Middle cerebral arteries
     C. Proximal carotid arteries
     D. Venous vessels

12. Typical peak velocities of the *ascending aorta* are usually within what range?
     A. 150 - 175 cm/sec
     B. 100 - 160 cm/sec
     C. 80 - 120 cm/sec
     D. 40 - 70 cm/sec

13. Typical peak velocities of the *distal aorta* and *iliac vessels* are usually within what range?
     A. 150 - 175 cm/sec
     B. 100 - 160 cm/sec
     C. 80 - 120 cm/sec
     D. 40 - 70 cm/sec

14. Typical peak velocities of the *proximal carotid, brachial* and *superficial femoral arteries* are usually within what range?
     A. 150 - 175 cm/sec
     B. 100 - 160 cm/sec
     C. 80 - 120 cm/sec
     D. 40 - 70 cm/sec

15. Typical peak velocities of the *middle and anterior cerebral arteries* are usually within what range?
     A. 150 - 175 cm/sec
     B. 100 - 150 cm/sec
     C. 40 - 70 cm/sec
     D. 30 - 50 cm/sec

11.d 12.a 13.b 14.c 15.c

16. Typical peak velocities of the vertebral and basilar arteries are usually within what range?
    A. 80-120 cm/sec
    B. 50-70 cm/sec
    C. 30-50 cm/sec
    D. under 20 cm/sec

17. The speed at which blood flows through an excited slice and only receives one RF pulse is known as what type of phenomenon?
    A. Time of flight phenomenon
    B. Entry slice phenomenon
    C. Intra-voxel dephasing
    D. None of the above

18. To produce signal in a spin echo pulse sequence, blood flow must receive both the 90 degree and the 180 degree RF pulse.
    A. True
    B. False

19. Blood flow that receives a 90 degree excitation pulse but not a 180 degree rephasing pulse produces what type of signal?
    A. High signal
    B. Low signal
    C. No signal

20. Blood flow that receives a 180 degree rephasing pulse but not a 90 degree excitation pulse produces what type of signal?
    A. High signal
    B. Low signal
    C. No signal

16.c 17.a 18.a 19.c 20.c

21. The magnitude of time of flight phenomenon effects is dependent upon which factor(s)?
    A. Velocity of flow
    B. TE
    C. Slice thickness
    D. All of the above

22. As blood flow velocity increases, the effects of time of flight phenomenon
    _____.
    A. Increase
    B. Decrease
    C. Stay the same

23. As blood flow velocity decreases, the effects of time of flight phenomenon
    _____.
    A. Increase
    B. Decrease
    C. Stay the same

24. As the echo time increases, the effects of time of flight phenomenon _____.
    A. Increase
    B. Decrease
    C. Stay the same

25. As echo time decreases, the effects of time of flight phenomenon _____.
    A. Increase
    B. Decrease
    C. Stay the same

26. As slice thickness increases, the effects of time of flight phenomenon _____.
    A. Increase
    B. Decrease
    C. Stay the same

21.d 22.a 23.b 24.a 25.b 26.b

27. As slice thickness decreases, the effects of time of flight phenomenon
_____.
    A. Increase
    B. Decrease
    C. Stay the same

28. In a gradient echo pulse sequence, blood flow that receives the initial RF pulse produces what type of signal?
    A. High
    B. Low
    C. No signal

29. The flow phenomenon that is characterized by the contrast differences between fresh flowing nuclei entering a slice and stationary tissue within that slice is known as _____.
    A. Time of flight phenomenon
    B. Entry slice phenomenon
    C. Intra-voxel dephasing
    D. None of the above

30. Entry slice phenomenon is most prominent in what slice of the area scanned?
    A. First slice
    B. Middle slice
    C. Last slice
    D. Affects all the same

31. The effects of entry slice phenomenon are dependent upon which factor(s)?
    A. Repetition time
    B. Slice thickness
    C. Velocity of flow
    D. All of the above

27.a 28.a 29.b 30.a 31.d

32. When TR is decreased, the effects of entry slice phenomenon _____.
    A. Increase
    B. Decrease
    C. Stay the same

33. When TR is increased, the effects of entry slice phenomenon _____.
    A. Increase
    B. Decrease
    C. Stay the same

34. When slice thickness is increased, the effects of entry slice phenomenon

    _____.
    A. Increase
    B. Decrease
    C. Stay the same

35. When slice thickness is decreased, the effects of entry slice phenomenon

    _____.
    A. Increase
    B. Decrease
    C. Stay the same

36. When the velocity of flow increases, the effects of entry slice phenomenon

    _____.
    A. Increase
    B. Decrease
    C. Stay the same

37. When the velocity of flow decreases, the effects of entry slice phenomenon

    _____.
    A. Increase
    B. Decrease
    C. Stay the same

32.b 33.a 34.b 35.a 36.a 37.b

38. The direction of blood flow is an important factor in determining the effects of entry slice phenomenon.
    A. True
    B. False

39. Blood flow that travels in the same direction in which the slices are acquired is known as what type of flow?
    A. Counter current flow
    B. Vortex flow
    C. Stagnant flow
    D. Co-current flow

40. Blood flow that travels in the opposite direction in which the slices are acquired is known as what type of flow ?
    A. Counter current flow
    B. Vortex flow
    C. Stagnant flow
    D. Co-current flow

41. When the direction of blood flow is opposite the direction in which slices are acquired, the effects of entry slice phenomenon _____.
    A. Increase
    B. Decrease
    C. Stay the same

42. When the direction of blood flow is the same as the direction in which slices are acquired, the effects of entry slice phenomenon _____.
    A. Increase
    B. Decrease
    C. Stay the same

38.a 39.d 40.a 41.a 42.b

43. The flow phenomenon that is characterized by phase differences between flowing and stationary nuclei within a voxel is known as _____.
    A. Time of flight phenomenon
    B. Entry slice phenomenon
    C. Intra-voxel dephasing
    D. None of the above

44. The magnitude of intra-voxel dephasing is dependent upon which factor(s)?
    A. Degree of disruption in the flow (ie degree of Turbulence)
    B. Echo time
    C. Repetition time
    D. None of the above

45. In which of the following types of flow can intra-voxel dephasing be compensated for?
    A. Turbulent flow
    B. Vortex flow
    C. Stagnant flow
    D. Laminar flow

46. The use of an additional gradient to correct the effects of intra-voxel dephasing is a technique known as _____.
    A. Gradient moment rephasing
    B. Intra-voxel misregistration
    C. Gradient moment nulling
    D. Both A and C

47. Gradient moment nulling is most effective on which type of flow?
    A. Slow turbulent flow
    B. Fast laminar flow
    C. Slow laminar flow
    D. Fast vortex flow

43.c 44.a 45.d 46.d 47.c

48. The effects of time of flight and entry slice phenomena can be minimized by which method?
    A. Gradient moment nulling
    B. Pre-saturation RF pulse
    C. Respiratory compensation
    D. None of the above

49. The method of acquiring more than one echo that are multiples of each other to reduce intra-voxel dephasing is known as _____.
    A. Gradient moment nulling
    B. Pre-saturation RF pulse
    C. Even echo rephasing
    D. None of the above

50. Which of the following conventional MRI techniques can be used to produce contrast differences between vascular structures and stationary structures?
    A. Gradient moment nulling
    B. Respiratory compensation
    C. Pre-saturation pulse
    D. Both A and C

51. Which of the following is the conventional technique used to produce a black appearance in vascular structures?
    A. Short TE, Short TR, Pre-saturation pulse
    B. Long TE, Short TR, Gradient moment nulling
    C. Long TE, Long TR, Respiratory compensation
    D. None of the above

52. Which of the following is the conventional technique used to produce a bright appearance in vascular structures?
    A. Pre-saturation pulse
    B. Respiratory compensation
    C. Gradient moment nulling
    D. None of the above

48.b 49.c 50d 51a 52c

53. The vascular imaging method that maximizes vascular contrast while also suppressing stationary tissue is known as _____.
    A. Magnetic resonance mammography
    B. Magnetic resonance angiography
    C. Black Blood imaging
    D. Zeugmatography

54. Which of the following is a method used in MRA to suppress stationary tissue?
    A. Tissue subtraction
    B. Tissue saturation
    C. Gradient moment nulling
    D. Both A and B

55. Which of the following is a method used in MRA to increase signal from vascular structures?
    A. Gradient moment nulling
    B. Subtraction
    C. Bipolar gradient
    D. Both A and C

56. The type of MRA that uses gradient echo pulse sequences and gradient moment nulling to enhance flow is known as _____.
    A. Digital subtraction
    B. TOF MRA
    C. PC MRA
    D. Velocity encoding

57. In TOF MRA, which method is used to suppress signal from stationary tissue?
    A. Saturation
    B. Subtraction
    C. Gradient moment nulling
    D. None of the above

53.b 54.d 55.d 56.b 57.a

58. TOF MRA is most sensitive to blood flow that flows in what direction in relation to the slice?
    A. Parallel
    B. Perpendicular

59. Which of the following is a disadvantage of TOF MRA?
    A. Parallel flow can be suppressed
    B. Slow flow can be suppressed
    C. Stationary tissue with short T1 relaxation times can produce signal
    D. All of the above

60. Which of the following is an advantage of TOF MRA?
    A. Relatively short scan times
    B. Increased sensitivity to flow
    C. Decreased sensitivity to intra-voxel dephasing
    D. All of the above

61. Which of the following TOF MRA sequences is most likely to saturate slow flow?
    A. 3D TOF
    B. 2D TOF

62. The type of MRA that produces image contrast based on the differences in phase shifts between blood flow and stationary tissue is known as _____.
    A. TOF MRA
    B. Velocity encoding
    C. PC MRA
    D. None of the above

58.b 59.d 60.d 61.a 62.c

63. Which of the following type of MRA uses a bipolar gradient to enhance vascular structures?
    A. TOF MRA
    B. Bright blood imaging
    C. Phase contrast MRA
    D. Black Blood imaging

64. Which of the following is a type of image that is produced by phase contrast MRA?
    A. Magnitude image
    B. Frequency image
    C. Phase image
    D. Both A and C

65. Which of the following is an advantage of phase contrast MRA?
    A. Increased stationary tissue suppression
    B. Sensitive to flow in all directions
    C. Sensitive to flow with various velocities
    D. All of the above

66. Which of the following is a disadvantage of phase contrast MRA?
    A. Long scan times
    B. Reduced intra-voxel dephasing
    C. Increased sensitivity to turbulence
    D. Both A and C

67. Which of the following PC MRA techniques provides the highest signal to noise ratio and spacial resolution?
    A. 2D PC MRA
    B. 3D PC MRA

63.c 64.d 65.d 66.d 67.b

68. The method that is most commonly used to reduce artifact produced by cardiac motion when scanning the chest is known as _____.
    A. Respiratory gating
    B. Respiratory compensation
    C. Cardiac gating
    D. None of the above

69. Two types of cardiac gating that are most commonly used are known as _____.
    A. Respiratory gating, Respiratory compensation
    B. ECG gating, Peripheral gating
    C. Pseudo gating, Respiratory gating
    D. None of the above

70. The P wave of the ECG represents which phase of the cardiac cycle?
    A. Atrial systole
    B. Ventricular systole
    C. Ventricular diastole
    D. Atrial diastole

71. The QRS wave of the ECG represents which phase of the cardiac cycle?
    A. Atrial systole
    B. Ventricular systole
    C. Ventricular diastole
    D. Atrial diastole

72. The T wave of the ECG represents which phase of the cardiac cycle?
    A. Atrial systole
    B. Ventricular systole
    C. Ventricular diastole
    D. Atrial diastole

68.c 69.b 70.a 71.b 72.c

73. During cardiac gating, which wave is used to trigger each pulse sequence?
    A. P wave
    B. Q wave
    C. R wave
    D. T wave

74. During cardiac gating, the time between two consecutive R waves is known
    as _____.
    A. Trigger window
    B. Trigger delay
    C. R-R interval
    D. None of the above

75. The ECG wave with the highest electrical amplitude is known as the _____.
    A. R wave
    B. Q wave
    C. T wave
    D. P wave

76. During cardiac gating, TR is dependent upon which factor(s)?
    A. The patient's heart rate
    B. The R- R interval
    C. The Q - R interval
    D. Both A and B

77. During cardiac gating, which factors are affected by having an effective TR?
    A. Image weighting
    B. Number of slices
    C. Scan time
    D. All of the above

73.c 74.c 75.a 76.d 77.d

78. During cardiac gating, the waiting time between the R wave and the start of the data acquisition is known as _____.
    A. Repetition time
    B. Inversion time
    C. Trigger delay
    D. Echo delay

79. During cardiac gating, the waiting time before each R wave is known as _____.
    A. Repetition time
    B. Inversion time
    C. Trigger delay
    D. Trigger window

80. During cardiac gating, which of the following is the formula used to calculate available imaging time?
    A. $F = \gamma B_o$
    B. Time = R-R interval - (trigger window + trigger delay)
    C. Time = R-R interval + (trigger window + trigger delay)
    D. None of the above

81. The type of cardiac gating that detects the increase in blood volume in the capillary bed during systole is known as _____.
    A. ECG gating
    B. Pseudo gating
    C. Peripheral gating
    D. None of the above

82. During cardiac gating, one R-R interval and a short TE is used to produce what type of image?
    A. T1 weighting
    B. T2 weighting
    C. Proton density weighting
    D. None of the above

78.c 79.d 80.b 81.c 82.a

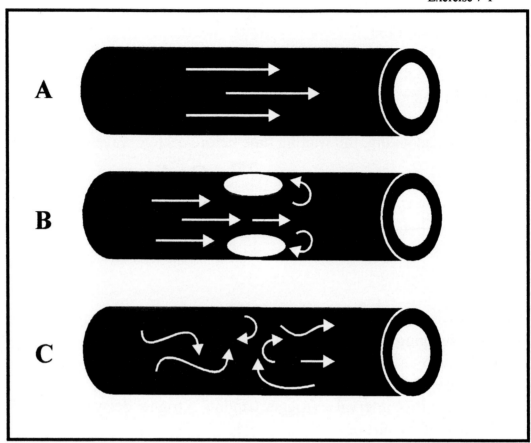

Using the correct answers to questions 1 through 4, label each type of flow.

A _____

B _____

C _____

SECTION 8

Instrumentation

Magnets
Gradients
Coils
Cryogens
Prescan

1. Which of the following is an advantage of a permanent magnet MRI system?
    A. Very heavy
    B. Low operating costs
    C. Fixed field strength
    D. Limited field strength

2. Which of the following types of MRI magnet is known as the *Classical* electromagnet?
    A. Resistive magnet
    B. Superconducting magnet
    C. Permanent magnet
    D. Distractive magnet

3. Which of the following is a disadvantage of a resistive magnet MRI system?
    A. Easy coil maintenance
    B. Low cost
    C. High power consumption
    D. None of the above

4. The type of MRI magnet that is produced by cooling a current down to 4 degrees Kelvin is known as a _____.
    A. Distractive magnet
    B. Permanent magnet
    C. Resistive magnet
    D. Superconducting magnet

5. The type of MRI magnet that allows the highest field strengths is a _____.
    A. Resistive magnet
    B. Superconducting magnet
    C. Iron core magnet
    D. Permanent magnet

6. Coils used to correct imperfections in the magnetic field are known as _____.
    A. RF coils
    B. Surface coils
    C. Gradient coils
    D. Shim coils

1.b 2.a 3.c 4.d 5.b 6.d

7. The type of magnet that is produced by permanently magnetizing a ferromagnetic substance is known as a_____.
    A. Resistive magnet
    B. Electromagnet
    C. Superconducting magnet
    D. Permanent magnet

8. In clinical MRI, permanent magnets can be produced to operate up to what field strength?
    A. .3 tesla
    B. .5 tesla
    C. 1.0 tesla
    D. 1.5 tesla

9. Which of the following is a disadvantage of using a permanent magnet in clinical MRI?
    A. Low fringe field
    B. Low operating cost
    C. Low field strength
    D. Both A and B

10. Which of the following materials is most commonly used to produce a permanent magnet ?
    A. Niobium-Titanium alloy
    B. Copper-Gadolinium alloy
    C. Aluminum-Nickel-Cobalt alloy
    D. Iron

11. The type of magnet that is produced by passing an electrical current through a conductor is known as a _____.
    A. Permanent magnet
    B. Resistive magnet
    C. Electromagnet
    D. Both B and C

7.d 8.a 9.c 10.c 11.d

12. The rule that is used to determine the direction of the magnetic field in an electromagnet is known as _____.
    A. Ohm's Law
    B. Right hand thumb rule
    C. Left hand thumb rule
    D. None of the above

13. In clinical MRI, resistive magnets usually operate at what field strength?
    A. Between 0.15 - .25 tesla
    B. Between .5 - 1.5 tesla
    C. Between 1.5 - 2 tesla
    D. Over 2 tesla

14. Which of the following is an advantage of using a resistive magnet for clinical MRI ?
    A. High power consumption
    B. Low capital cost
    C. Low field strength
    D. None of the above

15. The law that is used to determine the amount of resistance in a conductor is known as _____.
    A. Newton's Law
    B. Ohm's Law
    C. Faraday's Law
    D. Murphy's Law

16. The type of magnet that is produced by removing resistance from a conductive wire is known as _____.
    A. Resistive magnet
    B. Reactive magnet
    C. Permanent magnet
    D. Superconducting magnet

12.b 13.a 14.b 15.b 16.d

17. The wire used to create the main magnetic field in a superconducting magnet is known as _____.
    A. Aluminum-Tiobium
    B. Iron Sulfite
    C. Copper-Tungsten
    D. Niobium-Titanium

18. The external magnetic field in a superconducting magnet is said to be what type of magnetic field?
    A. Static
    B. Kinetic
    C. Gradient
    D. Resistive

19. The wire used in the main magnetic field of a superconducting magnet has its resistance removed by cooling it to a temperature of _____.
    A. -452 degrees Fahrenheit
    B. 0 degrees Celsius
    C. 269 degrees Kelvin
    D. None of the above

20. The liquids used to cool the wire in the main magnetic field of a superconducting magnet are known as _____.
    A. Neon gases
    B. Plasma
    C. Cryogens
    D. None of the above

21. The specific liquids used to maintain low temperatures in the superconducting wire are _____.
    A. Titanium and Niobium
    B. Hydrogen and Neon
    C. Halon and Oxygen
    D. Helium and Nitrogen

17.d 18.a 19.a 20.c 21.d

22. The device used to store and transport cryogenic liquids is known as a _____.
    A. Thermos
    B. Dewar
    C. Barrel
    D. None of the above

23. In a superconducting magnet, the sudden loss of superconductivity is known as a _____.
    A. Squelch
    B. Slouch
    C. Screech
    D. Quench

24. In an MRI system, the magnetic field that extends outside the bore of the magnet is known as the _____.
    A. Extended field
    B. Outer field
    C. Fringe field
    D. In field

25. In clinical MRI, superconducting magnets usually operate at field strengths from _____.
    A. .15 to .3 tesla
    B. .5 to 2.0 tesla
    C. 2.5 to 4.0 tesla
    D. Over 4 tesla

26. In clinical MRI, which of the following is an advantage of using a superconducting magnet?
    A. High field strength
    B. Shorter scan times
    C. Low power consumption
    D. All of the above

22.b 23.d 24.c 25.b 26.d

27. In clinical MRI, which of the following is a disadvantage of using a superconducting magnet?
    A. High capital costs
    B. High fringe field
    C. High cryogenic costs
    D. All of the above

28. The method used to contain the main magnetic field within the scan room is known as _____.
    A. Shimming
    B. Shielding
    C. Fringing
    D. None of the above

29. The method of MRI field containment that uses steel lining in the walls of the magnetic room is known as _____.
    A. Active shimming
    B. Passive shielding
    C. Active shielding
    D. Passive shimming

30. The method of MRI field containment that uses additional magnets outside the cryogenic area of the magnet is known as _____.
    A. Active shimming
    B. Passive shielding
    C. Active shielding
    D. Passive shimming

31. The process of adjusting coils to improve the homogeneity of the external magnetic field is known as _____.
    A. Strengthening
    B. Fringing
    C. Shielding
    D. Shimming

27.d 28.b 29.b 30.c 31.d

32. Each shim coil requires its own power supply.
    A. True
    B. False

33. The type of shimming that is achieved by placing a ferrous material around the main magnet is known as _____.
    A. Passive shimming
    B. Passive shielding
    C. Active shimming
    D. Active shielding

34. The type of shimming that is achieved by adjusting the electrical current in specialized coils is known as _____.
    A. Passive shimming
    B. Passive shielding
    C. Active shimming
    D. Active shielding

35. The homogeneity of the external magnetic field is measured in what type of unit?
    A. Tesla per centimeter
    B. Part per million
    C. Gauss per meter
    D. Megahertz

36. In clinical MRI, the homogeneity of the magnet should be at least _____.
    A. 1 tesla per cm
    B. 10 parts per million
    C. .5 gauss per meter
    D. 32 megahertz

32.a 33.a 34.c 35.b 36.b

37. The type of coils used to change the strength of the magnetic field inside the bore of the magnet are known as _____.
    A. RF coils
    B. Shim coils
    C. Surface coils
    D. Gradient coils

38. In a gradient coil, the amplitude of the gradient slope is determined by what factor?
    A. The amount of current passing through the coil
    B. Transmit bandwidth
    C. The strength of the external magnetic field
    D. None of the above

39. How many gradient coils are there in a clinical MRI system?
    A. 1 pair
    B. 2 pairs
    C. 3 pairs
    D. 4 pairs

40. Gradient strength is measured in what form of unit?
    A. Megahertz
    B. Gauss per centimeter
    C. Millitesla per meter
    D. Both B and C

41. The time it takes for a gradient coil to reach its peak strength is known as its _____.
    A. Repetition time
    B. Echo time
    C. Rise time
    D. Inversion time

37.d 38.a 39.c 40.d 41.c

42. Coils that are used to transmit and receive radio frequencies are known as
_____.
    A. RF coils
    B. Shim coils
    C. Gradient coils
    D. Surface coils

43. The type of RF coil that encompasses the entire anatomy to be scanned is
known as _____.
    A. Surface coil
    B. Phased array coil
    C. Volume coil
    D. Gradient coil

44. The type of RF coil configuration that uses a pair of coils perpendicular to
each other to transmit and receive signal is known as a _____.
    A. Surface coil
    B. Phased array coil
    C. Quadrature coil
    D. Shim coil

45. The type of RF coil configuration that uses a series of independent coils to
create one image is known as a _____.
    A. Surface coil
    B. Phased array coil
    C. Quadrature coil
    D. Gradient coil

46. The type of RF coil configuration that is used to image anatomical structures
close to the surface of the patient is known as a _____.
    A. Surface coil
    B. Quadrature coil
    C. Phased array coil
    D. Shim coil

42.a 43.c 44.c 45.b 46.a

47. Mutual induction between the RF transmitter and the RF receiver is known as _____.
    A. Isolation
    B. Deisolation
    C. Coupling
    D. Decoupling

48. Isolating the RF transmitter from the RF receiver is known as _____.
    A. Deisolation
    B. Isolation
    C. Coupling
    D. Decoupling

49. The computer that performs the complex calculations necessary to reconstruct MRI images is known as the _____.
    A. Array processor
    B. RF amplifier
    C. Gradient amplifier
    D. Shim cabinet

50. The device in the MRI system that supplies power to the gradient coils is known as the _____.
    A. Array processor
    B. RF amplifier
    C. Gradient amplifier
    D. None of the above

51. The device in the MRI system that supplies power to the RF transmitter coils is known as the _____.
    A. Array processor
    B. RF amplifier
    C. Gradient amplifier
    D. None of the above

47.c 48.d 49.a 50.c 51.b

52. Prior to each scan, the process of prescanning performs which type of calibration?
    A. Adjusts the transmit gain
    B. Adjusts the receive attenuation
    C. Sets the center frequency
    D. All of the above

53. The calibration of *transmit gain* during the prescan process determines which factor?
    A. RF output necessary to produce a 90 degree flip angle
    B. The exact resonant frequency
    C. The necessary amount of signal needed to create an image
    D. None of the above

54. The process during the prescan that determines the amount of signal that is received is known as _____.
    A. Center frequency adjustment
    B. Transmit gain adjustment
    C. Receive attenuation adjustment
    D. Impedance matching

55. The process during prescan that fine tunes the resonant frequency is known as _____.
    A. Center frequency adjustment
    B. Transmit gain adjustment
    C. Receive attenuation adjustment
    D. Impedance matching

56. How many miliseconds are there in a minute?
    A. 60
    B. 600
    C. 6,000
    D. 60,000

52.d 53.a 54.c 55a 56.d

Figure 8-1

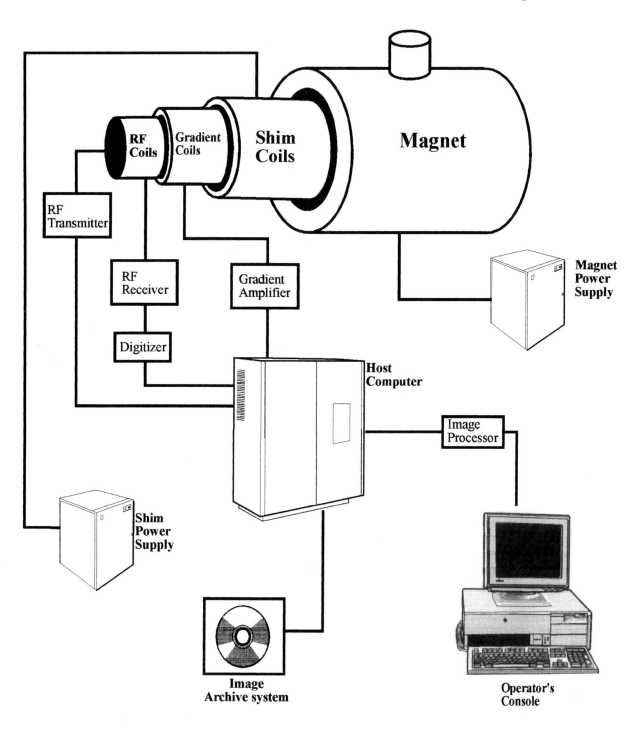

SECTION 9

Safety
Biological Effects
Contrast Media

Patient Screening
Patient Monitoring
Safety Precautions
Static Magnetic Fields
Radio Frequency
Gradient Magnetic Fields
Relaxivity
Administration
Application
Side Effects

1. Thorough patient preparation should include which of the following?
   A. Proper patient screening
   B. Complete patient medical history
   C. Adequate patient education
   D. All of the above

2. Proper patient screening should include which of the following?
   A. The elimination of any loose metal objects and personal items
   B. The identification of any possible contraindications
   C. The identification of any biomedical implants
   D. All of the above

3. Complete medical history should include which of the following?
   A. Patient age, sex, and weight
   B. Current physical symptoms
   C. Previous surgeries and associated medical problems
   D. All of the above

4. Adequate patient education should include which of the following?
   A. Thorough description of the procedure
   B. Complete physics review
   C. The importance of remaining still
   D. Both A and C

5. Ancillary equipment that should be excluded from the magnetic room includes which of the following?
   A. Ferrous oxygen tanks
   B. Battery powered IV pumps
   C. Ferrous scissors, pens and hemostats
   D. All of the above

1.d 2.d 3.d 4.d 5.d

6. Ancillary equipment that should be included in an MRI department includes which of the following?
   A. Non-ferrous wheelchair or stretcher
   B. Proper monitoring equipment for sedated patients
   C. A crash cart for emergency situations
   D. All of the above

7. Which of the following ancillary staff should be trained in the safety procedures of the MRI department?
   A. Janitorial staff
   B. Nursing staff
   C. MRI department clerical staff
   D. All of the above

8. Which of the following pieces of equipment should be used and or available when sedating patients for an MRI examination?
   A. Pulse oximeter
   B. Blood pressure monitor
   C. Crash cart
   D. All of the above

9. Which of the following patient injuries can be caused by improper placement of cardiac leads?
   A. Patient burns
   B. Temporary hearing loss
   C. Short term memory loss
   D. None of the above

10. RF coils should be looped during scanning to improve signal to noise.
    A. True
    B. False

6.d 7.d 8.d 9.a 10.b

11. Which of the following is an important environmental consideration necessary to maintain proper computer and gradient function?
    A. Temperature
    B. Barometric pressure
    C. Humidity
    D. Both A and C

12. Which of the following objects should not be permitted past the 5 gauss line?
    A. Cardiac pacemaker
    B. Hearing aids
    C. Neuro stimulators
    D. All of the above

13. Which of the following objects will be affected by a magnetic field of 10 gauss or higher?
    A. Video cameras
    B. Monitors
    C. Cameras
    D. All of the above

14. Metal implants within the body, depending on the location, can pose what type of problems during the MRI exam?
    A. Torque
    B. Heating
    C. Artifacts
    D. All of the above

15. Hazards to patients and technologists due to ferromagnetic objects within the scan room include which of the following?
    A. Metal projectiles
    B. Tissue burns
    C. Image artifacts
    D. None of the above

11.d 12.d 13.d 14.d 15.a

16. The force on a ferromagnetic object placed in a magnetic field is dependent upon which of the following factors?
    A. The mass of the object
    B. The distance from the magnet
    C. The object's orientation to the magnet
    D. All of the above

17. Which of the following patients should be absolutely excluded from having an MRI exam?
    A. Patients with hip replacements
    B. Patients with titanium aneurysm clips
    C. Patients with cardiac pacemakers
    D. Patients with cornea implants

18. Which of the following patients should be monitored with a pulse oximeter during an MRI procedure?
    A. Sedated patients
    B. Unconscious patients
    C. Patients with weak voices or hearing problems
    D. All of the above

19. Which of the following hazards can occur due to an improperly ventilated quench?
    A. Frostbite due to decrease room temperature
    B. Hearing loss due to increased air pressure in the scan room
    C. Patient suffocation due to loss of oxygen
    D. All of the above

20. The magnetic field that surrounds the Earth has what field strength?
    A. .5 tesla
    B. .6 tesla
    C. .5 gauss
    D. 1.5 tesla

16.d 17.c 18.d 19.d 20.c

21. Biological effects associated with exposure to static magnetic fields *below* 2 tesla include which of the following?
    A. Increased amplitude at the T wave on an EKG
    B. Nausea and vomiting
    C. Minimal increase in body temperature
    D. Both A and C

22. Biological effects associated with exposure to static magnetic fields *above* 2 tesla include which of the following?
    A. Fatigue
    B. Headaches
    C. Hypotension
    D. All of the above

23. Possible biological effects associated with exposure to gradient magnetic fields at levels higher than that used in MRI include which of the following?
    A. Voltage produced in conductive tissue
    B. Hypertension
    C. Tissue burns
    D. None of the above

24. Biological effects associated with exposure to radio frequency include which of the following?
    A. Induction of electrical currents in tissue
    B. Heating due to tissue resistance
    C. Radiation poisoning
    D. Both A and B

25. The rate at which a patient can safely dissipate excess heat caused by RF energy is known as_____.
    A. Specific absorption time
    B. Specific absorption rate
    C. Signal absorption rate
    D. None of the above

21.d 22.d 23.a 24.d 25.b

26. Specific absorption rate is expressed in units of what?
    A. Watts/kg
    B. Ohms/kg
    C. Amps/kg
    D. Watts/lb

27. Heating that is directly associated with the RF pulse sequence should not increase the core body temperature greater than _____.
    A. 1 degree Fahrenheit
    B. 1 degree Kelvin
    C. 10 degrees Celsius
    D. 1 degree Celsius

28. Which of the following is a biological effect unique to echo planar imaging?
    A. Visual phosphenes
    B. Muscular twitches in face and back
    C. Tissue burns
    D. None of the above

29. Specific absorption rate is dependent upon which factor(s)?
    A. Induced electrical field and tissue density
    B. Patient size and pulse duty cycle
    C. Tissue conductivity
    D. All of the above

30. The recommended whole body SAR limit for MR imaging is_____.
    A. .4 Watts/kg
    B. 3.2 Watts/kg
    C. 8 Watts/kg
    D. 4.0 Watts/kg

26.a 27.d 28.b 29.d 30.a

31. The recommended SAR limit for safely imaging the head is _____.
    A. .4 Watts/kg
    B. 3.2 Watts/kg
    C. 8 Watts/kg
    D. 4.0 Watts/kg

32. The recommended SAR limit for safely imaging small volumes is_____.
    A. .4 Watts/kg
    B. 3.2 Watts/kg
    C. 8 Watts/kg
    D. 4.0 Watts/kg

33. The effect of MRI contrast media on tissue relaxation rates is known as

    _____.
    A. Relaxation
    B. Relaxivity
    C. Realization
    D. None of the above

34. Contrast agents presently used in MRI have what type of effect on tissue?
    A. Increase T2 relaxation times
    B. Decrease T1 relaxation times
    C. Increase T1 relaxation times
    D. None of the above

35. The first material used by Felix Bloch to change magnetic relaxation times was
    known as _____.
    A. Niobium-Titanium
    B. Gadopentetate dimeglumine
    C. Ferric Nitrate
    D. Nickel-Cadmium

31.b 32.c 33.b 34.b 35.c

36. The first use of a paramagnetic agent on a human subject was in what year?
    A. 1976
    B. 1981
    C. 1946
    D. 1973

37. The first oral MRI contrast agent used in a human subject was known as
    _____.
    A. Niobium-Titanium
    B. Ferric Chloride
    C. Ferric Nitrate
    D. Gadopentetate dimeglumine

38. The first intravenous MRI contrast agent that was used on a human subject
    was known as _____.
    A. Niobium-Titanium
    B. Ferric Chloride
    C. Ferric Nitrate
    D. Gadopentetate dimeglumine

39. Gadolinium has how many unpaired electrons in its outermost orbit?
    A. 5
    B. 7
    C. 9
    D. 11

40. MRI contrast agents known as T1 agents produce what type of contrast
    on T1 weighted images?
    A. Positive
    B. Negative

41. MRI contrast agents known as T2 agents produce what type of contrast
    on T2 weighted images?
    A. Positive
    B. Negative

36.b 37.b 38.d 39.b 40.a 41.b

42. MRI contrast agents known as T2 agents have what type of effect on tissue?
    A. Increase T2 relaxation times
    B. Increase T1 relaxation times
    C. Decrease T2 relaxation times
    D. None of the above

43. Which of the following is a requirement for a chemical before it can be used as an MRI contrast medium?
    A. It must decrease magnetic relaxation times
    B. Must be non-ionic
    C. Must be biologically compatible with the human body
    D. Both A and C

44. The chemical compounds used to bind the metallic ion in MRI contrast agents are known as _____.
    A. Hydrophilies
    B. Chelates
    C. Macrophanges
    D. None of the above

45. To minimize MRI contrast agent's toxicity, the agent should be _____.
    A. Excreted intact by the kidneys
    B. Excreted intact by the gallbladder and intestines
    C. Released within the body
    D. Both A and B

46. The amount of a drug required to cause death in half of a sample of laboratory mice is known as _____.
    A. LD50
    B. LR50
    C. Median lethal dose
    D. Both A and C

42.c 43.d 44.b 45.d 46.d

47. Which of the following is the median lethal dose of Gadopentetate dimeglumine?
    A. .5 mmol/kg
    B. 5 mmol/kg
    C. 1 mmol/kg
    D. 10-20 mmol/kg

48. Contrast agents that stay electrically neutral in water and do not separate into ions are said to be _____ .
    A. Hydrophilic
    B. Nonionic
    C. Ionic
    D. None of the above

49. Contrast agents that separate into charged ions in water are said to be _____ .
    A. Hydrophobic
    B. Nonionic
    C. Ionic
    D. None of the above

50. The diffusion of fluid thorough a semipermeable membrane such as the wall of a living cell is known as _____ .
    A. Hydrosis
    B. Ionization
    C. Osmosis
    D. None of the above

51. The osmolality of a contrast agent is measured in what unit?
    A. Osmoles per kilogram of water (Osm/kg)
    B. Milliosmoles per kilogram of water (mOsm/kg)
    C. Milliliters per kiloliter (ml/kl)
    D. Both A and B

47.d 48.b 49.c 50.c 51.d

52. The effective clinical dosage of gadolinium is how many millimoles per kilogram of body weight?
    A. 1.0 mmol/kg
    B. 0.1 mmol/kg
    C. 10 mmol/kg
    D. 20 mmol/kg

53. Which of the following is a possible side effect of gadopentetate dimeglumine?
    A. Mild, temporary headaches
    B. Nausea
    C. Vomiting
    D. All of the above

54. Gd DTPA, also known as Magnevist, is bound by which chelate?
    A. Bismethylamide
    B. Diethylenetriamine pentaacetic acid
    C. Tertraazacyclododecane tetraacetic acid
    D. None of the above

55. Gd DOTA, also known as Dotarem, is bound by what chelate?
    A. Bismethylamide
    B. Diethylenetriamine pentaacetic acid
    C. Tertraazacyclododecane tetraacetic acid
    D. None of the above

56. Gd DTPA-BMA, also known as Omniscan, is bound by what chelate?
    A. Bismethylamide
    B. Diethylenetriamine pentaacetic acid
    C. Tertraazacyclododecane tetraacetic acid
    D. None of the above

52.b 53.d 54.b 55.c 56.a

57. Gadoteridol, also known as ProHance, is based on what type of molecular structure?
    A. Linear ionic
    B. Linear nonionic
    C. Macrocyclic ionic
    D. Macrocyclic nonionic

58. Gadopentetate dimeglumine, also known as Magnevist, is based on what type of molecular structure?
    A. Linear ionic
    B. Linear nonionic
    C. Macrocyclic ionic
    D. Macrocyclic nonionic

59. Gadodiamide, also known as Omniscan, is based on what type of molecular structure?
    A. Linear ionic
    B. Linear nonionic
    C. Macrocyclic ionic
    D. Macrocyclic nonionic

60. Gadoterate meglumine, also known as Dotarem, is based on what type of molecular structure?
    A. Linear ionic
    B. Linear nonionic
    C. Macrocyclic ionic
    D. Macrocyclic nonionic

61. Which of the following is a clinical indication for the use of MRI contrast agents?
    A. CNS tumors
    B. Post surgical lumbar discs
    C. Infection
    D. All of the above

57.d 58.a 59.b 60.c 61.d

62. Structures that are outside the blood brain barrier are said to be _____.
    A. Extra axial
    B. Intra axial
    C. Para axial
    D. None of the above

63. The type of neoplasms in the head that enhance primarily due to their increase in vascularity are known as _____.
    A. Intra axial neoplasms
    B. Extra axial neoplasms
    C. Metastatic neoplasms
    D. None of the above

64. Which of the following is an example of an extra axial neoplasm?
    A. Meningioma
    B. Astrocytoma
    C. Acoustic Neuroma
    D. Both A and C

65. The type of neoplasms in the head that enhance primarily due to the breakdown of the blood brain barrier are known as _____.
    A. Intra axial neoplasms
    B. Extra axial neoplasms
    C. Acoustic neuromas
    D. None of the above

66. Which of the following is an example of an intra axial neoplasm?
    A. Acoustic neuroma
    B. Meningioma
    C. Astrocytoma
    D. Both A and B

62.a 63.b 64.d 65.a 66.c

67. Which area outside the blood brain barrier shows normal enhancement with the injection of gadolinium?
    A. Choroid plexus
    B. Pineal gland
    C. Pituitary gland
    D. All of the above

68. Which of the following is an example of a non-neoplastic disease of the brain that enhances with the injection of gadolinium?
    A. Meningitis
    B. Demyelinating disease
    C. Cerebral infection
    D. All of the above

69. Neoplasms within the spinal cord are said to be located in which of the following locations?
    A. Intramedullary
    B. Extramedullary Intradural
    C. Extradural
    D. None of the above

70. Neoplasms outside the spinal cord but within the CSF space are said to be located in which of the following locations?
    A. Intramedullary
    B. Extramedullary Intradural
    C. Extradural
    D. None of the above

71. Neoplasms of the spine that are outside the spinal cord and outside the CSF space are said to be located in which of the following locations?
    A. Intramedullary
    B. Extramedullary Intradural
    C. Extradural
    D. None of the above

67.d 68.d 69.a 70.b 71.c

72. Which of the following pathologies of the spine is an indication for the use of an MRI contrast agent?
    A. Spinal cord infection
    B. Recurrent disc herniation
    C. Intramedullary neoplasm
    D. All of the above

73. Which of the following is a *contraindication* for the use of gadolinium?
    A. Patients with history of metastatic cancer
    B. Patients with history of asthma
    C. Patients with history of metal implants
    D. No known contraindications

74. Which of the following is a *precaution* for the use of gadolinium?
    A. Patients with sickle cell anemia
    B. Patients with a history of grand mal seizures
    C. Patients with a history of asthma
    D. All of the above

72.d 73.d 74.d

Draw a line to match the brand name and the structure type to the diagram of the contrast agent.

ProHance
Macrocyclic Nonionic

Gadopentetate dimeglumine

Magnevist
Linear Ionic

Gadodiamide

Omniscan
Linear Nonionic

Gadoterate meglumine

Dotarem
Macrocyclic Ionic

Gadoteridol

SECTION 10

Cross Sectional Anatomy

Brain
Spine
Shoulder
Knee
Chest
Abdomen
Pelvis
Heart
Arteries
Circle of Willis/
Aortic Arch/Carotids

1. _____
2. _____
3. _____
4. _____
5. _____
6. _____
7. _____
8. _____
9. _____
10. _____
11. _____
12. _____
13. _____
14. _____
15. _____
16. _____

A. Fourth ventricle
B. Pituitary gland
C. Cerebellum
D. Clivus
E. Cerebrum
F. Quadrigeminal body
G. Pons
H. Lateral ventricle
I. Medulla oblongata
J. Sphenoid sinus
K. Optic chiasm
L. Corpus callosum (genu)
M. Corpus callosum (splenium)
N. C-2
O. Thalamus
P. Cerebral peduncle

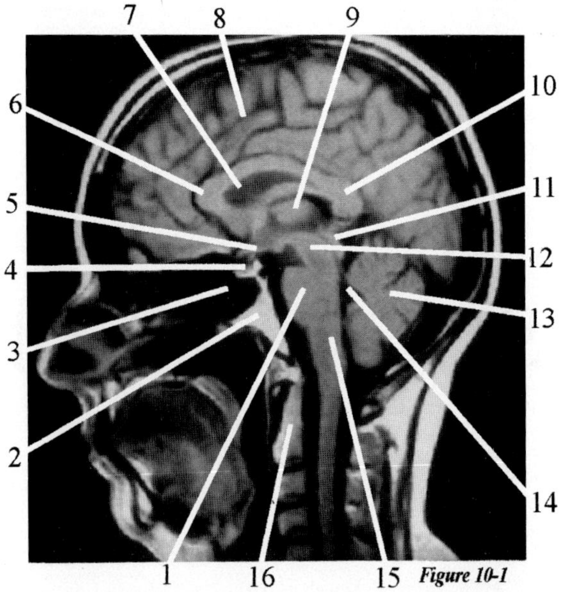

Figure 10-1

17. _____
18. _____
19. _____
20. _____
21. _____
22. _____
23. _____
24. _____
25. _____
26. _____

Q. Internal capsule
R. Lentiform nucleus
S. Superior sagittal sinus
T. Head of caudate nucleus
U. Thalamus
V. External capsule
W. Corpus callosum
X. Frontal lobe
Y. Occipital lobe
Z. Interhemispheric fissure

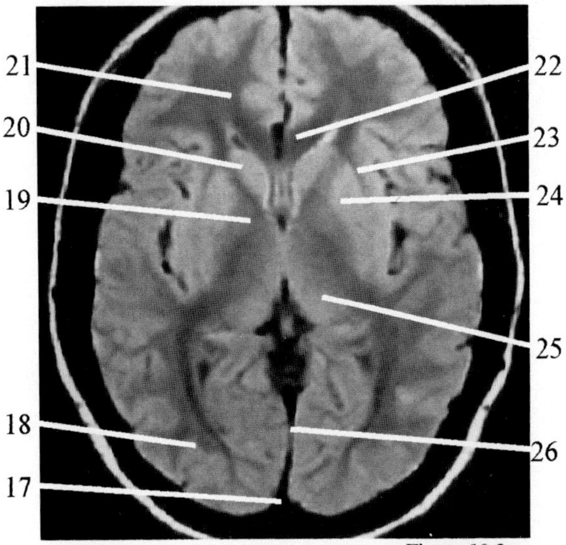

Figure 10-2

27. _____
28. _____
29. _____
30. _____
31. _____
32. _____
33. _____
34. _____
35. _____
36. _____

AA. Third ventricle
BB. Septum pellucidum
CC. Superior sagittal sinus
DD. Thalamus
EE. Lateral ventricle
FF. Temporal lobe
GG. Sylvian fissure
HH. Pons
II. Petrous ridge
JJ. Corpus callosum

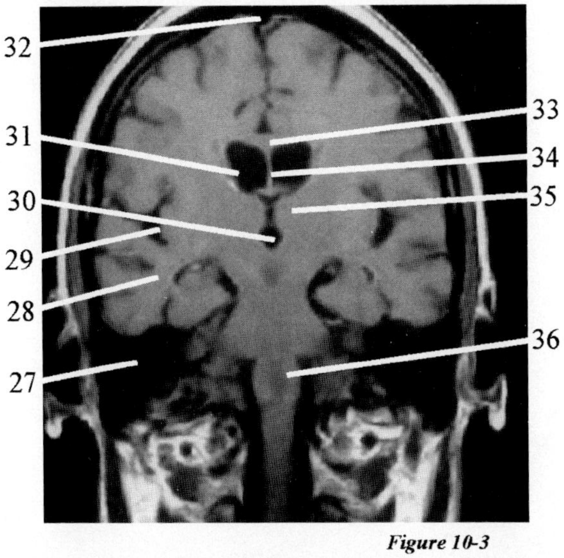

Figure 10-3

1. _____
2. _____
3. _____
4. _____
5. _____
6. _____
7. _____
8. _____
9. _____
10. _____

A. Intervertebral disk
B. Cerebellum
C. Trachea
D. Vertebral body C-5
F. Medulla oblongata
G. Cervical cord
H. CSF
I. Epiglottis
J. Vertebral body T-1
K. Spinous process

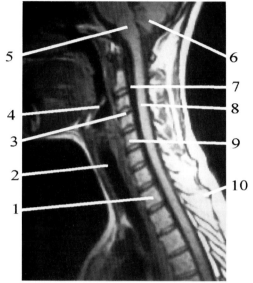

Figure 10-4

11. _____
12. _____
13. _____
14. _____
15. _____
16. _____
17. _____

L. Jugular vein
M. Vertebral body
N. Trachea
O. Facet joint
P. Cervical cord
Q. CSF
R. Carotid artery

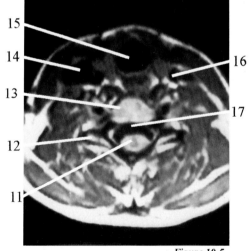

Figure 10-5

1. _____   A. Spinous process
2. _____   B. CSF
3. _____   C. Intervertebral disk
4. _____   D. Vertebral body
5. _____   E. Thoracic spinal cord

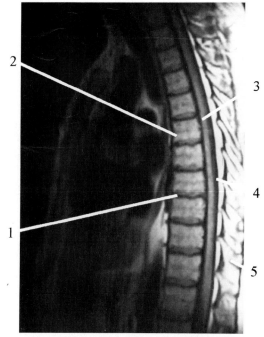

Figure 10-6

6. _____   F. Vertebral body
7. _____   G. Abdominal aorta
8. _____   H. Rib
9. _____   I. Lamina
10. _____   J. Spinal cord
11. _____   K. Pedicle
12. _____   L. CSF

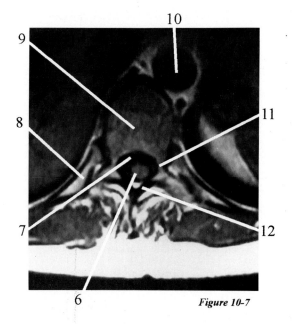

Figure 10-7

1. _____
2. _____
3. _____
4. _____
5. _____
6. _____
7. _____

A. Spinous process
B. CSF
C. Conus medularis
D. Intervertebral disk
E. S1 vertebra
F. L5 vertebra
G. Intracanal fat

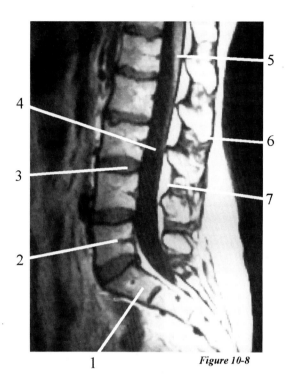

Figure 10-8

8. _____
9. _____
10. _____
11. _____
12. _____
13. _____
14. _____
15. _____

H. Iliac aorta
I. Lamina
J. Pedicle
K. CSF
L. Facet joint
M. Vertebral body
N. Spinous process
O. Psoas muscle

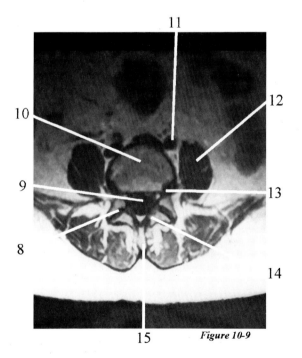

Figure 10-9

1. _____
2. _____
3. _____
4. _____
5. _____
6. _____

A. Supraspinatus muscle
B. Acromion process
C. Rotator cuff
D. Lateral deltoid muscle
E. Glenoid
F. Humerus

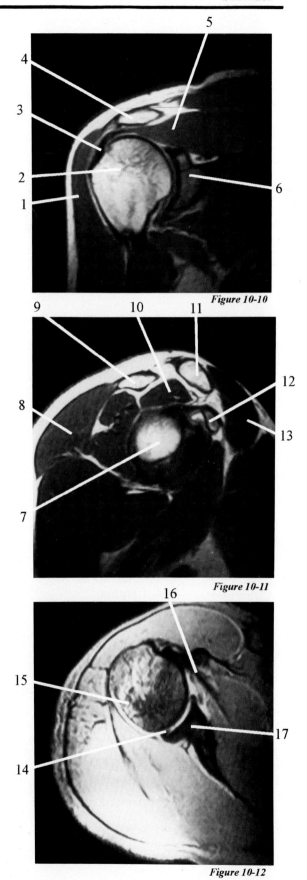

Figure 10-10

7. _____
8. _____
9. _____
10. _____
11. _____
12. _____
13. _____

G. Acromion process
H. Coracoid process
I. Supraspinatus muscle
J. Humerus
K. Posterior deltoid muscle
L. Anterior deltoid muscle
M. Clavicle

Figure 10-11

14. _____
15. _____
16. _____
17. _____

N. Humerus
O. Biceps tendon
P. Glenoid
Q. Glenoid labrum

Figure 10-12

Figure 10-13

1. _____
2. _____
3. _____
4. _____
5. _____
6. _____
7. _____
8. _____
9. _____

A. Anterior cruciate ligament
B. Posterior cruciate ligament
C. Patella
D. Femur
E. Quadriceps tendon
F. Patellar tendon
G. Tibia
H. Infrapatellar fat
I. Gastrocnemius muscle

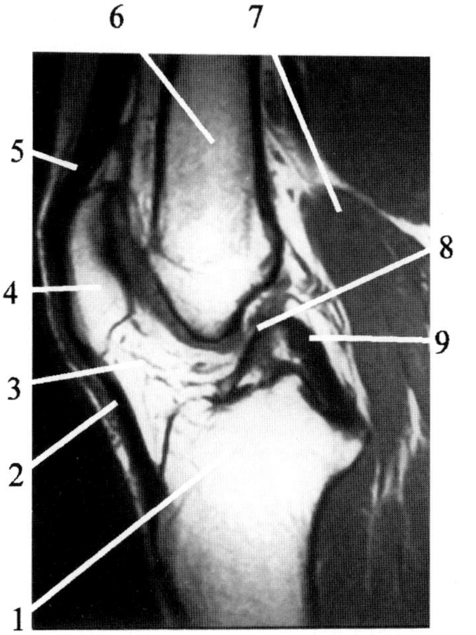

Figure 10-14

10. _____
11. _____
12. _____
13. _____
14. _____

J. Patella
K. Femoral condyle
L. Femoral biceps muscle
M. Patellar ligament
N. Popliteal artery

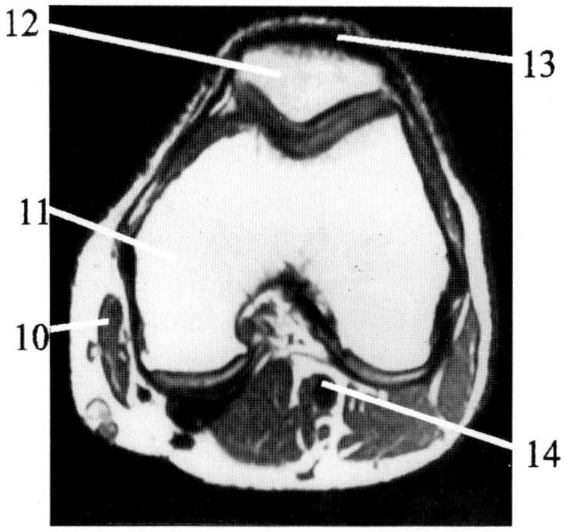

Figure 10-15

15. _____
16. _____
17. _____
18. _____
19. _____
20. _____
21. _____
22. _____
23. _____
24. _____

O. Popliteal artery
P. Lateral femoral condyle
Q. Medial meniscus
R. Fibula
S. Tibia
T. Medial collateral ligament
U. Lateral meniscus
V. Anterior cruciate ligament
W. Posterior cruciate ligament
X. Medial femoral condyle

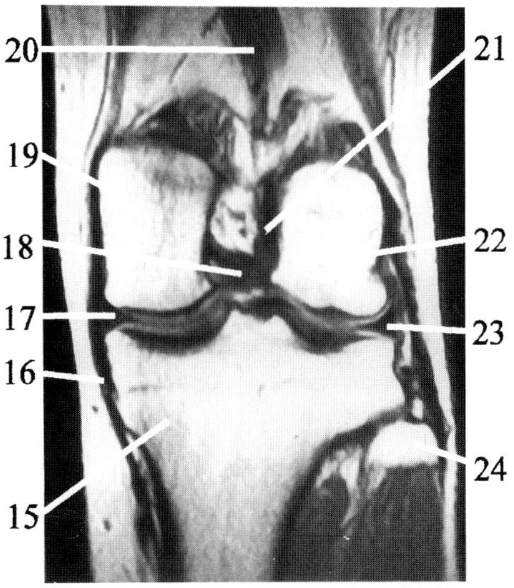

1. _____
2. _____
3. _____
4. _____
5. _____
6. _____
7. _____
8. _____
9. _____

A. Cervical spine
B. Left ventricle
C. Stomach
D. Liver
E. Aortic arch
F. Pulmonary artery
G. Lung
H. Trachea
I. Right atrium

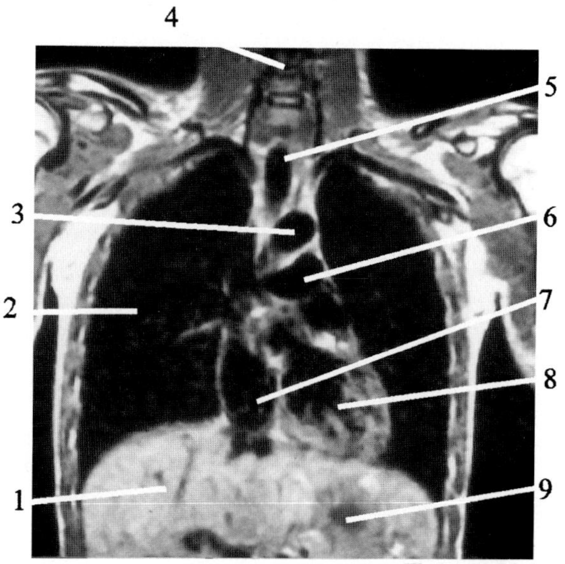

Figure 10-16

10. _____
11. _____
12. _____
13. _____
14. _____
15. _____
16. _____
17. _____
18. _____

J. Ascending aorta
K. Right pulmonary artery
L. Lung
M. Vertebral body
N. Spinal cord
O. Left pulmonary artery
P. Main pulmonary artery
Q. Descending aorta
R. Superior vena cava

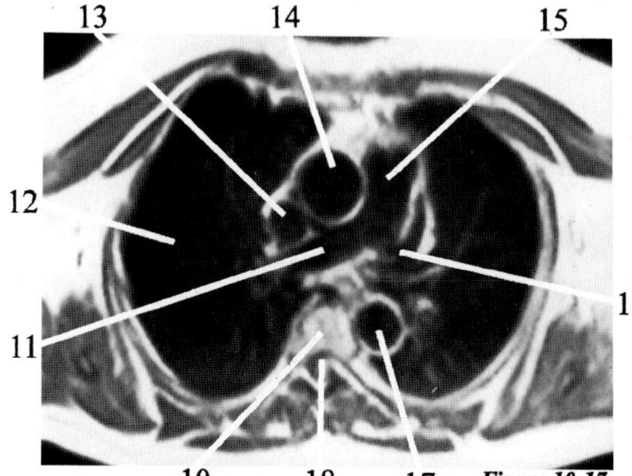

Figure 10-17

19. _____
20. _____
21. _____
22. _____
23. _____
24. _____
25. _____
26. _____

S. Carotid artery
T. Descending aorta
U. Sternum
V. Liver
W. Main pulmonary artery
X. Right ventricle
Y. Left atrium
Z. Left subclavian artery

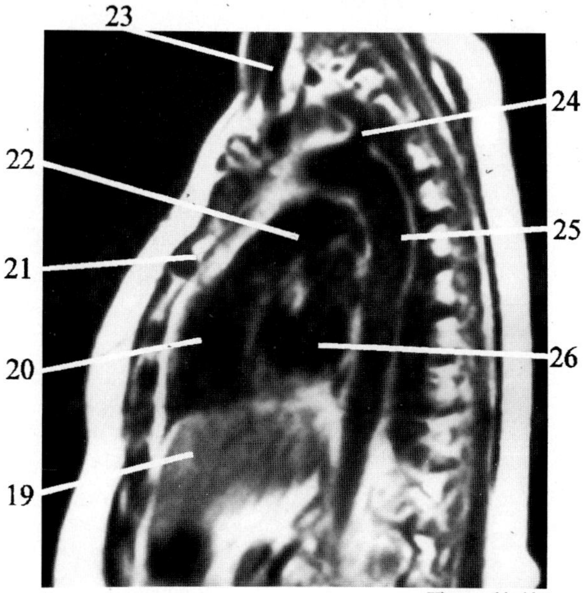

Figure 10-18

1. _____
2. _____
3. _____
4. _____
5. _____
6. _____
7. _____
8. _____
9. _____

A. Descending aorta
B. Left psoas muscle
C. Lumbar vertebrae
D. Right kidney
E. Thoracic vertebrae
F. Liver
G. Spleen
H. Left lung
I. Iliac crest

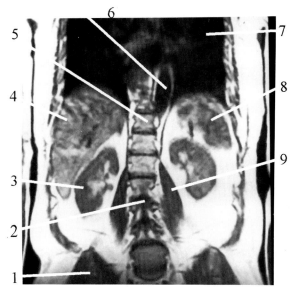

Figure 10-19

10. _____
11. _____
12. _____
13. _____
14. _____
15. _____
16. _____
17. _____
18. _____

J. Portal vein
K. Liver
M. Right kidney
N. Vertebral body
O. Stomach
P. Abdominal aorta
Q. Inverior vena cava
R. Spleen
S. Pancreas

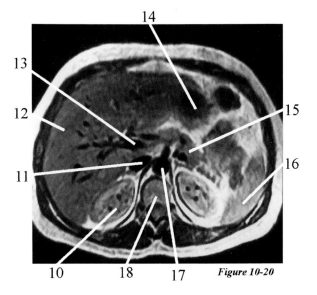

Figure 10-20

1. _____   A. Sacrum
2. _____   B. Right femoral head
3. _____   C. Left ilium
4. _____   D. Sacral iliac joint
5. _____   E. Ovary
6. _____   F. Right acetabulum
7. _____   G. Vagina
8. _____   H. Uterus
9. _____   I. Bowel
10. _____   J. Left femoral head

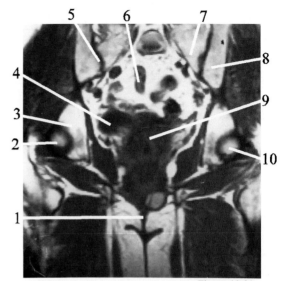

Figure 10-21

11. _____   K. Rectum
12. _____   L. Bladder
13. _____   M. Right femoral head
14. _____   N. Left acetabulum
15. _____   O. Fovea capitis

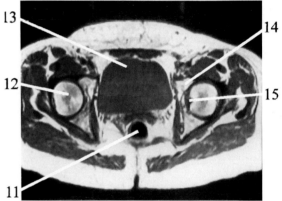

Figure 10-22

16. _____   P. Sacrum
17. _____   Q. Lumbar vertebra
18. _____   R. Uterus
19. _____   S. Bladder
20. _____   T. Pubic bone
21. _____   U. Rectum
22. _____   V. Colon
23. _____   W. Vagina

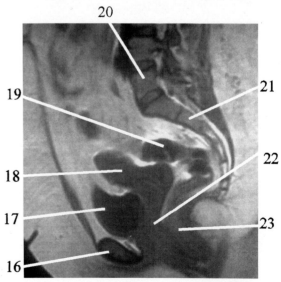

Figure 10-23

Figure 10-24

1. _____   A. Left psoas muscle
2. _____   B. Bladder
3. _____   C. Right femoral head
4. _____   D. Prostate gland
5. _____   E. Left acetabulum
6. _____   F. Right femur
7. _____   G. Right ilium

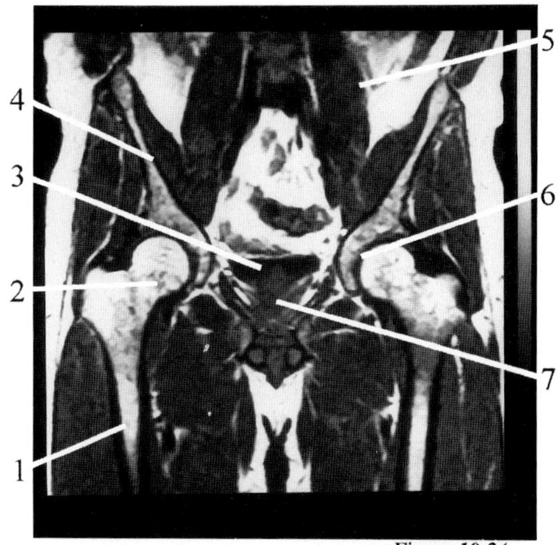

Figure 10-25

8. _____   H. Bladder
9. _____   I. Rectum
10. _____   J. Right femoral head
11. _____   K. Left femoral artery & vein
12. _____   L. Left posterior acetabulum

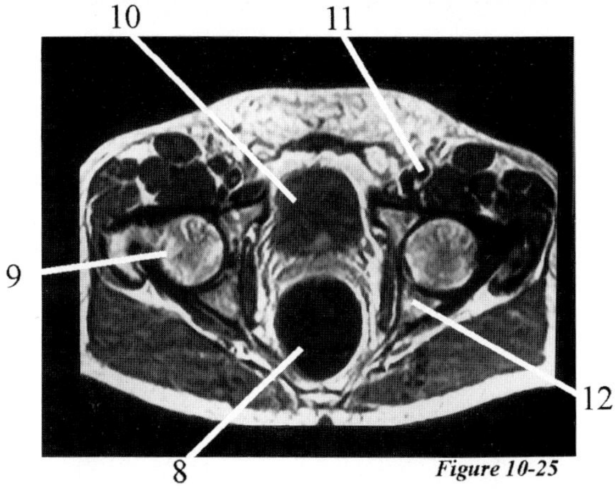

Figure 10-26

13. _____   M. Sacrum
14. _____   N. Prostate gland
15. _____   O. Pubis
16. _____   P. Testis
17. _____   Q. Bladder
18. _____   R. Urethra
19. _____   S. Penis
20. _____   T. Rectum
21. _____   U. Seminal vesicles
22. _____   V. Anus

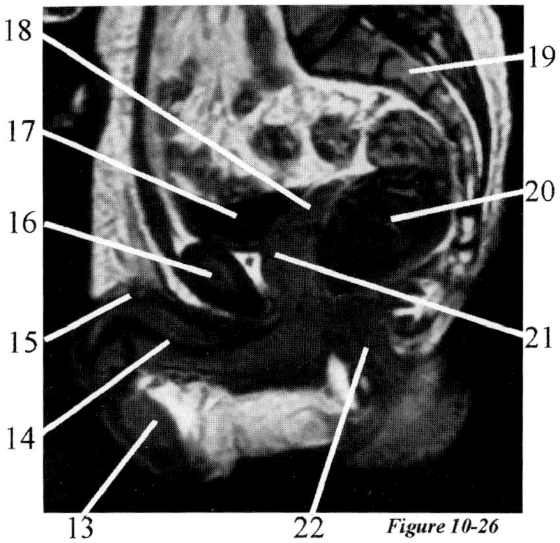

1. _____   A. Descending aorta
2. _____   B. Left atrium
3. _____   C. Right atrium
4. _____   D. Superior vena cava
5. _____   E. Right pulmonary veins
6. _____   F. Left ventricle
7. _____   G. Right ventricle
8. _____   H. Left pulmonary veins
9. _____   I. Ascending aorta
10. _____   J. Inferior vena cava
11. _____   K. Interventricular septum
12. _____   L. Left common carotid artery
13. _____   M. Left subclavian artery
14. _____   N. Left pulmonary artery

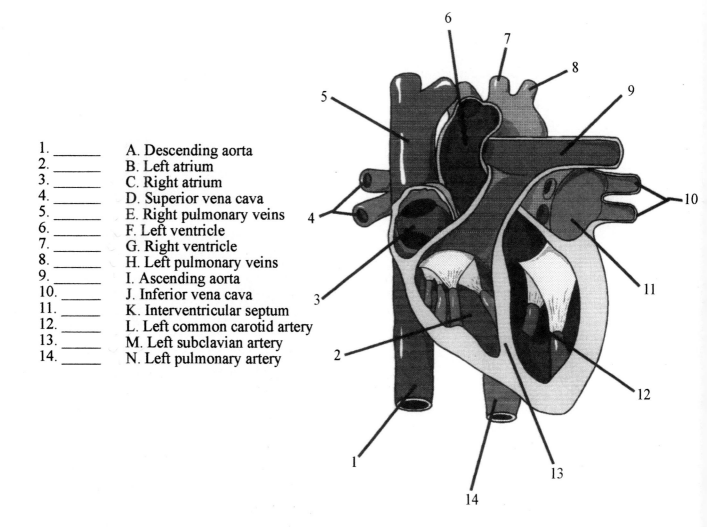

Figure 10-27

1. _____ A. Left commom carotid
2. _____ B. Right subclavian
3. _____ C. Left axillary
4. _____ D. Left common iliac
5. _____ E. Abdominal aorta
6. _____ F. Right renal
7. _____ G. Left internal iliac
8. _____ H. Right radial
9. _____ I. Right ulnar
10. _____ J. Right femoral
11. _____ K. Ascending aorta
12. _____ L. Celiac
13. _____ M. Left anterior tibial
14. _____ N. Right brachial

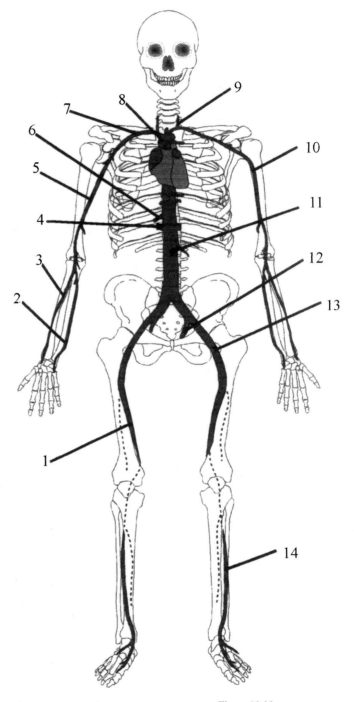

Figure 10-28

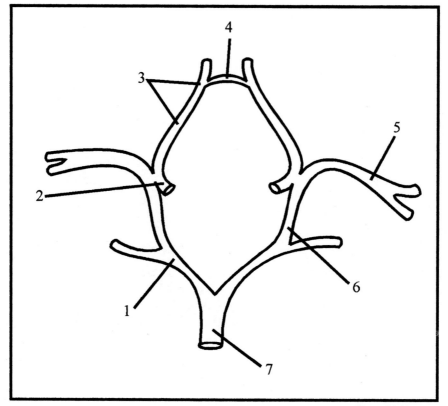

Figure 10-29

1. _____
2. _____
3. _____
4. _____
5. _____
6. _____
7. _____

A. Anterior communicating artery
B. Internal carotid artery
C. Middle cerebral artery
D. Anterior cerebral artery
E. Basilar artery
F. Posterior communicating artery
G. Posterior cerebral artery

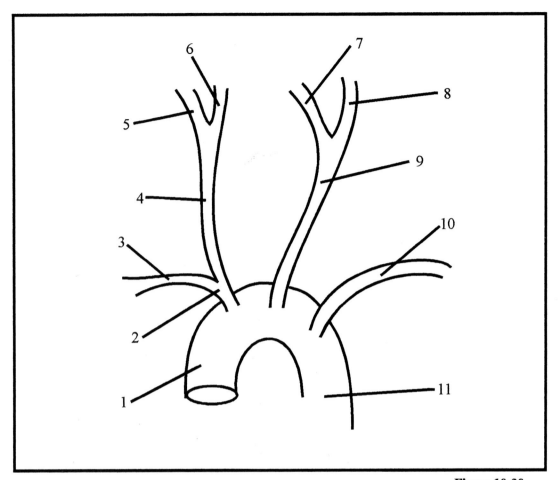

Figure 10-30

1. _____
2. _____
3. _____
4. _____
5. _____
6. _____
7. _____
8. _____
9. _____
10. _____
11. _____

A. Left subclavian
B. Left internal carotid
C. Right external carotid
D. Right subclavian
E. Descending aorta
F. Aortic arch
G. Right internal carotid
H. Left external carotid
I. Left carotid
J. Right carotid
K. Brachiocephalic

ANSWERS | Anatomy and Exercise

BRAIN

Figure 10-1	**Figure 10-2**	**Figure 10-3**
1. G	17. S	27. II
2. D	18. Y	28. FF
3. J	19. Q	29. GG
4. B	20. T	30. AA
5. K	21. X	31. EE
6. L	22. W	32. CC
7. H	23. V	33. JJ
8. E	24. R	34. BB
9. O	25. U	35. DD
10. M	26. Z	36. HH
11. F		
12. P		
13. C		
14. A		
15. I		
16. N		

CERVICAL SPINE

Figure 10-4	**Figure 10-5**
1. J	11. P
2. C	12. O
3. A	13. M
4. I	14. L
5. F	15. N
6. B	16. R
7. H	17. Q
8. G	
9. D	
10. K	

THORACIC SPINE

Figure 10-6	**Figure 10-7**
1. C	6. J
2. D	7. L
3. E	8. H
4. B	9. F
5. A	10. G
	11. K
	12. I

LUMBAR SPINE

Figure 10-8	**Figure 10-9**
1. E	8. L
2. F	9. K
3. D	10. M
4. B	11. H
5. C	12. O
6. A	13. J
7. G	14. I
	15. N

SHOULDER

Figure 10-10	**Figure 10-11**	**Figure 10-12**
1. D	7. J	14. Q
2. F	8. K	15. N
3. C	9. G	16. O
4. B	10. I	17. P
5. A	11. M	
6. E	12. H	
	13. L	

KNEE

Figure 10-13	**Figure 10-14**	**Figure 10-15**
1. G	10. L	15. S
2. F	11. K	16. T
3. H	12. J	17. Q
4. C	13. M	18. W
5. E	14. N	19. X
6. D		20. O
7. I		21. V
8. A		22. P
9. B		23. U
		24. R

CHEST

Figure 10-16	Figure 10-17	Figure 10-18
1. D	10. M	19. V
2. G	11. K	20. X
3. E	12. L	21. U
4. A	13. R	22. W
5. H	14. J	23. S
6. F	15. P	24. Z
7. I	16. O	25. T
8. B	17. Q	26. Y
9. C	18. N	

ABDOMEN

Figure 10-19	Figure 10-20
1. I	10. M
2. C	11. Q
3. D	12. K
4. F	13. J
5. E	14. O
6. A	15. S
7. H	16. R
8. G	17. P
9. B	18. N

FEMALE PELVIS

Figure 10-21	Figure 10-22	Figure 10-23
1. G	11. K	16. T
2. B	12. M	17. S
3. F	13. L	18. R
4. E	14. N	19. V
5. D	15. O	20. Q
6. I		21. P
7. A		22. W
8. C		23. U
9. H		
10. J		

MALE PELVIS

Figure 10-24	Figure 10-25	Figure 10-26
1. F	8. I	13. P
2. C	9. J	14. R
3. B	10. H	15. S
4. G	11. K	16. O
5. A	12. L	17. Q
6. E		18. U
7. D		19. M
		20. T
		21. N
		22. V

HEART

Figure 10-27
1. J
2. G
3. C
4. E
5. D
6. I
7. L
8. M
9. N
10. H
11. B
12. F
13. K
14. A

ARTERIES

Figure 10-28
1. J
2. I
3. H
4. F
5. N
6. L
7. B
8. K
9. A
10. C
11. E
12. G
13. D
14. M

CIRCLE OF WILLIS

Figure 10-29
1. G
2. B
3. D
4. A
5. C
6. F
7. E

AORTIC ARCH/CAROTIDS

Figure 10-30
1. F
2. K
3. D
4. J
5. C
6. G
7. B
8. H
9. I
10. A
11. E

Match the scientist with his contribution to MRI by placing the letter that corresponds to the scientist in the box next to his accomplishment.

A. Jean Baptiste Joseph Fourier   **E.** Felix Bloch

B. Michael Faraday   **F.** Edward Purcell

C. Niels Bohr   **G.** Paul Lauterbur

D. Nikola Tesla   **H.** Raymond Damadian

[E/F] Won the 1952 Nobel Prize for NMR research

[A] Developed the mathematical formula used to reconstruct images from signal

[B] Discovered the law of magnetic induction

[G] Described the imaging technique known as Zeugmatography

[C] Developed the theory of atomic structure

[H] Designed the first whole body NMR scanner for imaging

[D] Developed a method to generate alternating current and has a magnetic unit of measurement named after him

Exercise 2-1

A. __Electron__

B. __Proton__

C. __Neutron__

With the information given, label each atomic particle.

Exercise 2-2

Tesla	Gauss
.3	3,000
.5	5,000
1.0	10,000
1.5	15,000
2.0	20,000

Using the correct answer to question 15, convert each field strength from tesla to gauss.

Exercise 2-3

Field Strength	Gyromagnetic Ratio	Precessional Frequency
.3	42.6	12.78MHz
.5	42.6	21.3MHz
1.0	42.6	42.6MHz
1.5	42.6	63.9MHz
2.0	42.6	85.2MHz

Using the Larmor equation, calculate the precessional frequency of hydrogen at each field strength.

$$F = yBo$$

F = Precessional Frequency
y = Gyromagnetic Ratio
Bo = Field Strength

In section 3, using the correct answers to questions 38 through 59, fill in the tissue relaxation chart.

Approximate Relaxation Times
at 1.0 Tesla

Tissue	T1 time	T2 time
Fat	180ms	90ms
Liver	270ms	50ms
Renal cortex	360ms	70ms
White matter	390ms	90ms
Spleen	480ms	80ms
Grey matter	520ms	100ms
Muscle	600ms	40ms
Renal medulla	680ms	140ms
Blood	800ms	180ms
CSF	2000ms	300ms
Water	2500ms	2500ms

Exercise 4-1

Draw an arrow showing the effects that each parameter has on SNR, Spacial Resolution, and Scan Time.

Increase ↑ Decrease ↓	Signal to Noise Ratio	Spacial Resolution	Scan Time
↑ TR	↑	No Change	↑
↑ TE	↓	No Change	No Change
↓ NEX	↓	No Change	↓
↓ Matrix	↑	↓	↓
↑ Slice Thickness	↑	↓	No Change
↑ FOV	↑	↓	No Change
↓ Slice Gap	↓	No Change	No Change

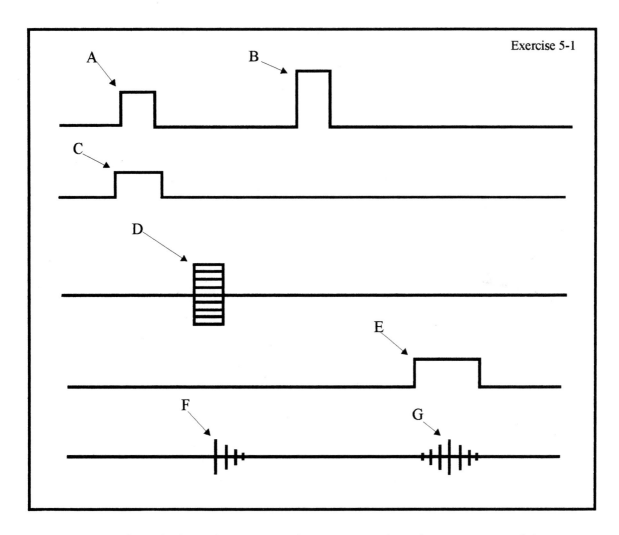

Exercise 5-1

Place the letter in the space that corresponds to the proper part of the pulse sequence.

<u>G</u>   Spin Echo Signal   <u>E</u>   Readout Gradient

<u>D</u>   Phase Encoding Gradient   <u>C</u>   Slice Select Gradient

<u>B</u>   180° Radio Frequency Pulse   <u>A</u>   90° Radio Frequency Pulse

<u>F</u>   FID Signal

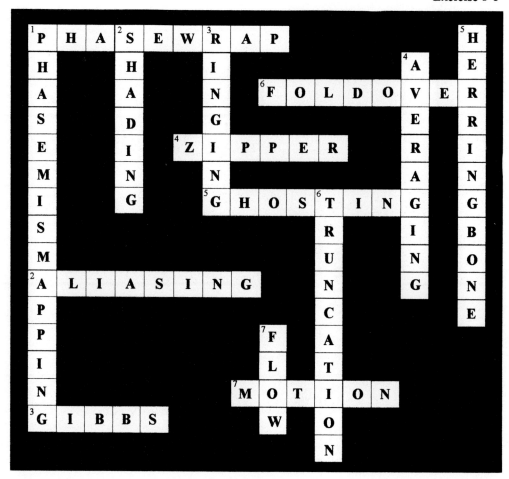

ACROSS

1. Another name for Aliasing artifact.

2. Another name for Foldover artifact.

3. Another name for Truncation artifact.

4. External RF artifact.

5. Respiratory motion artifact.

6. Another name for Phase Wrap artifact.

7. An artifact caused by an uncooperative patient.

DOWN

1. Another name for Ghosting artifact.

2. Artifact caused by inhomogeneity of the external magnetic field.

3. Another name for Gibbs artifact.

4. Volume _____.

5. Artifact named after a fish skeleton.

6. Another name for Ringing artifact.

7. Type of artifact caused by vascular structures.

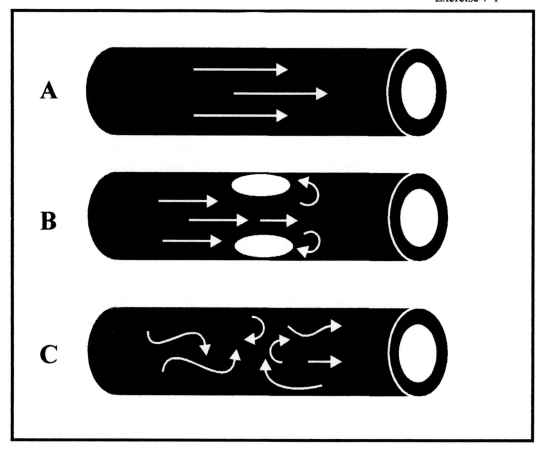

Using the correct answers to questions 1 through 4, label each type
of flow.

A   Laminar Flow

B   Vortex Flow

C   Turbulent Flow

Draw a line to match the brand name and the structure type to the diagram of the contrast agent.

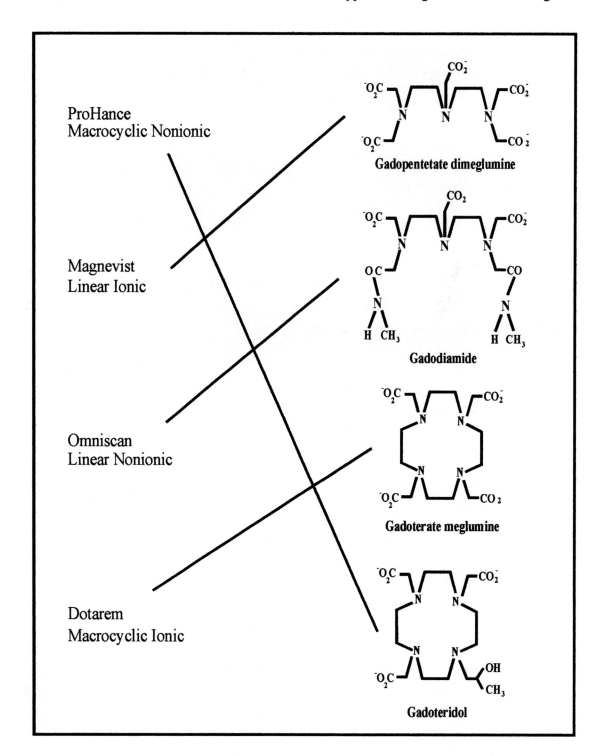

ProHance
Macrocyclic Nonionic

Magnevist
Linear Ionic

Omniscan
Linear Nonionic

Dotarem
Macrocyclic Ionic

Gadopentetate dimeglumine

Gadodiamide

Gadoterate meglumine

Gadoteridol

Bibliography

1. Applegate, Edith J. The Sectional Learning System. W.B. Saunders Company, Philadelphia, PA, 1992.

2. Berlex Laboratories Inc., MRI for Technologists. Competence Assurance Systems Inc.,1990.

3. Berquist, Thomas H. Ehman, Richard L. May, Gerald R. Pocket Atlas of MRI Body Anatomy. Raven Press, New York, NY, 1987.

4. Bushong, Stewart C. Magnetic Resonance Imaging Physical and Biological Principles. C.V. Mosby Company, St. Louis, MO, 1988.

5. Elster, Allen D. Questions and Answers in Magnetic Resonance Imaging. Mosby Yearbook Inc., St. Louis, MO, 1994.

6. General Medical Systems, Understanding Magnetic Resonance. GE Medical Systems, Milwaukee, WI, 1989.

7. Hole, John W., Jr. Human Anatomy and Physiology. Third Edition. Wm. C. Brown Publishers, Dubuque, IA, 1984.

8. Horowitz, Alfred L. MRI Physics for Radiologists: A Visual Approach. Second Edition, Springer-Verlag, New York, NY, 1992.

9. Kaut, Carolyn MRI Workbook For Technologists. Raven Press, New York, NY, 1992.

10. Liebman, Michael Neuroanatomy Made Easy and Understandable. Fourth Edition. Aspen Publishers, Inc., Gaithersburg, MD, 1991.

11. Lufkin, Robert B. The MRI Manual. Mosby Yearbook Inc. St. Louis, MO, 1990.

12. Schild, Hans H. MRI Made Easy ... Well Almost. Schering AG Berlin/Bergkaman, 1990.

13. Smith Hans-J., Ranallo, Frank N. A Non-Mathematical Approach to Basic MRI. Medical Physics Publishing Corporation, Madison, WI, 1989.

14. Westbrook, Catherine, Kaut, Carolyn MRI in Practice. Blackwell Scientific Publications, Oxford, England, 1993.

15. Young Stuart W. Nuclear Magnetic Resonance Imaging: Basic Principles. Raven Press, New York, NY, 1984.